BECOMING MINDSTRONG

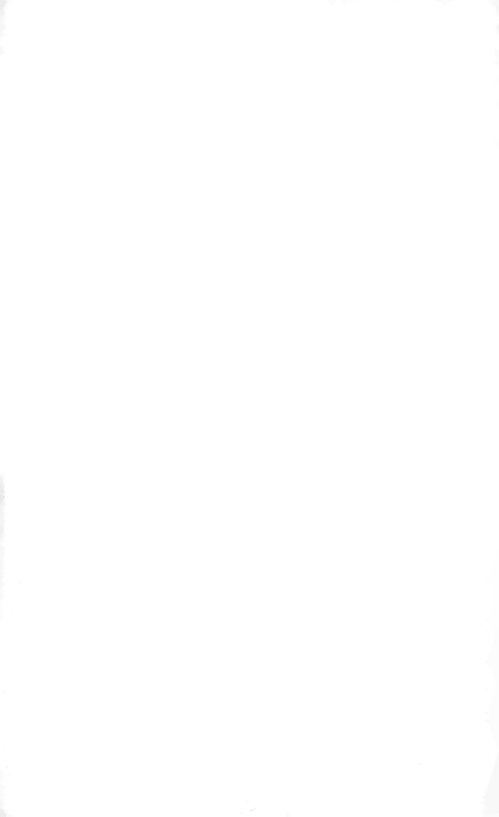

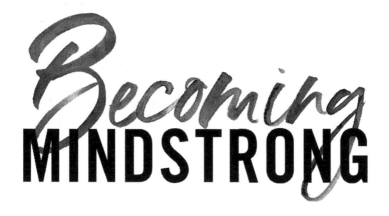

Becoming MINDSTRONG

The Truth About Health, Fitness, and
the Bullsh*t That's Holding You Back

RACHEL FREIMAN

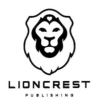

LIONCREST
PUBLISHING

BECOMING MINDSTRONG
*The Truth About Health, Fitness, and the
Bullsh*t That's Holding You Back*

ISBN   978-1-5445-1466-6 *Hardcover*
        978-1-5445-1465-9 *Paperback*
        978-1-5445-1464-2 *Ebook*

To Ellis,

My Gladiator-in-Training

CONTENTS

INTRODUCTION 9

1. WHERE TO START 17

2. THE BLUE GORILLA IN THE ROOM: RESTRICTION 35

3. MINDSET 51

4. THOUGHTS-FEELINGS-ACTIONS-RESULTS 73

5. A TRIP TO THE CREEPY FARMHOUSE: HABIT 107

6. REDEFINE FEAR 133

7. LIFE IS ENERGY 157

8. FAT LOSS: CALORIES IN VS. CALORIES OUT 177

9. INTRO TO MACROS.. 205

10. MACRO BREAKDOWN....................................... 233

11. DAY ONE 257

ADDITIONAL RESOURCES.............................. 269

ACKNOWLEDGMENTS................................... 271

ABOUT THE AUTHOR 273

REFERENCES 275

INTRODUCTION

THE BULLSHIT CUTTER-THROUGHER

"There is no passion to be found playing small—in settling for a life that is less than the one you are capable of living"
—NELSON MANDELA

JAZZ CLUBS, MIDDLE SCHOOL, AND FITNESS

There are certain things the world doesn't need more of:

- Variations on potato chips. Seriously, they make a grilled-cheese-and-ketchup-flavored chip. We've gone too far.
- Another generation of personal trainers showering you with spit while screaming in your face, "Pain is weakness leaving the body."
- Yet another quick-fix, fad diet that promises the world but doesn't deliver.

Which is exactly why I wrote this book.

I wasn't born into a lifestyle of fitness. I definitely wasn't one of those oddly buff ten-year-olds you see online, practically bench pressing their parents before they're out of elementary school.

In fact, my résumé reads more like someone smooshed the résumés of three different people into one long, random one.

I started out as a jazz trumpet player in New York City. Yes, growing up, I was a band nerd.

While playing gigs everywhere from main stages to hole-in-the-wall jazz clubs to sold-out Elvis impersonator concerts (true story) made for an exciting life, I eventually traded it in for a relatively calmer one of teaching middle school band in South Florida. I say calmer because compared to New York City jazz clubs at 2:00 a.m., a life full of middle school students seems like child's play, pun intended.

Relatively is the key word here. Teaching lacked the hustle-and-bustle of life as a freelance musician, but working with eleven-year-olds to thirteen-year-olds all day wasn't without its own challenges. Lifting heavy shit at the gym became my favorite way to let off steam. This is where my love of fitness was born.

As I learned and developed within my own health and fitness journey, I earned certifications in both personal training and sports nutrition. Through that education, and the consistent time and effort I put into my own training and nutrition, I became increasingly flabbergasted by the plethora of misinformation, money-making schemes, and flat-out bullshit that is sold as "truth" to consumers.

Listen, I'm an optimist. My brother, Jason, tells me that my love of the human race is nauseating at times. But even my glass-half-full outlook can't see past the fact that there is a ton of absolute crap on the market, packaged with a pretty pink bow and sold as the next magic pill to your current health woes. It broke my heart to see people I care about spend endless amounts of time and money, putting all their faith in *this* being the program that finally works, only to be disappointed yet again, reaffirming their belief that they'll never achieve their health and fitness goals.

So, I decided to do something different.

THE BIRTH OF MINDSTRONG FITNESS

I absolutely love teaching. Aside from the fact that my sense of humor is on par with that of a twelve-year-old, and that intense debates about how *obviously unlimited strength would be a way cooler superpower than flying* are high up on my list of passions, I especially love the moments where you can see your students "get it." You watch the switch flick on, the light bulb light up, their eyes brighten, and you know you've reached them. Those *aha!* moments are when you know you've made a difference in their lives, and that feeling is unparalleled.

Teaching had very little to do with the subject matter for me. It was about *life*. Middle school is a confusing time for kids, and helping to mold them into confident leaders and put them on a solid path is why I got into the profession. My students and I would talk about everything from dealing with adversity to *choosing* instead of *reacting*, the power of asking questions, and developing self-confidence.

As the school year would progress and our conversations were reinforced, I would begin to see changes in many of the kids. I saw the quiet ones speak up. I saw them gain the confidence to ask questions when they felt lost, despite being the only hand in the air. I heard their stories of how they chose a better reaction than indulging in gossip, which, shocking I know, runs rampant in middle school hallways.

I saw these kids starting to become strong, confident leaders.

Knowing that I could play a part in that and provide a safe place for them to come to when they needed guidance in making better choices lit me up.

It's where I discovered that my passion in life lies not in the teaching of a single subject matter but in helping people unleash the strongest, most empowered version of themselves.

This love of empowerment combined with my love of teaching created the perfect opportunity to educate, not only on the logistics of health and fitness but also on the mental and emotional side of health. My work in this world is to show you how to unleash your best life through a healthy body *and* a healthy mind. Not so you can *look* a certain way, but so you can *feel* a certain way. So you can show up as the strongest, most empowered, badass version of yourself for both you and those you love and have the *confidence* and *energy* to live a life that lights you up. *This* is where my company, MindStrong Fitness, was born.

As I immersed myself in the health and fitness world, I saw some huge gaps in the industry. There are two *vital* components to making this stuff stick, and I was hard-pressed to find anyone doing them:

1. **Education.** *Real* education. Not "here's how to follow our

program" but "here's how nutrition, exercise, and mindset work according to math, science, and human psychology." Here's not only *what* to do but *why it's working* so you can do it for the rest of your life.

2. **Mindset.** You can make all the physical changes you dream of, but if your mind is still telling you that *you're not worth it, it'll never last,* and *who are you kidding thinking you can change,* you're heading down a well-worn path called Self Sabotage Avenue. We all have deep-seated habits and beliefs that keep us in our comfort zone. It's only by first *identifying* them and then taking *conscious, consistent action* that we can make true, lasting change. This starts with training our mind along with our body and going about the process in a way that flows *with* our human nature, not against it.

It made complete sense why most fitness and nutrition companies avoided teaching this way. In an industry designed to keep consumers coming back, this was teaching a person to fish versus giving them a fish, setting people up with the tools they need for a sustainable lifestyle without needing you, your company, or anyone else. And, to most, that's just not smart business.

I believe in something bigger: human connection. I believe that when you go out in the world with the intention of helping as many people as possible, it is always the right choice.

So that's exactly what I set out to do.

I started MindStrong Fitness to teach *truth.* To show people that there are concrete rules to how nutrition and fitness work and you *can* learn them, no matter how many times you've started and stopped. I'm here to break through the bullshit and to educate.

To teach people how to *train their minds* along with their bodies, and to instill new, empowered habits that last a lifetime.

My role in life is not to spit in my clients' faces, demanding one more rep and insisting they eat nothing but chicken and vegetables three meals a day for the rest of their lives.

My role is an educator, a bullshit cutter-througher, a truth spreader, a coach, a best friend, an ass kicker when needed, and an accountability buddy. But the top of that list will always be educator.

This book isn't another fad diet. Or point system. Or self-help-think-your-way-thin book.

This is a book about what *true* health and fitness look like, both physical and mental. The *why* behind your current state and the *how* to get where you dream of going. The tools you need to live the empowered, healthy life you've always wanted and step-by-step instructions on how to apply these tools so that this becomes your new way of living. It's a sustainable approach to health and fitness that, when applied, will unleash your most empowered, energetic, badass life.

I will show you that you *can* absolutely do this no matter how many times you've started and stopped in the past and give you the tools to do exactly that.

We'll identify what's held you back in the past and break through those limiting beliefs to form new, healthy habits, both physically and mentally.

We'll walk through the process, step-by-step, until you feel confident to take it from there, indefinitely.

Throughout these pages, you'll find *actionable* steps to do all of this. This isn't some fluffy-feel-good-pump-you-up book of mantras. Within these pages are tools to both train your body *and* train your mind.

It works when you do the work.

It will take time to trust yourself on this journey. The good news is that you don't need to yet. I have enough trust in you for the both of us until you're ready to take the reins.

XO,
Rachel

CHAPTER I

WHERE TO START

"Jump off the cliff and build your wings on the way down."
—RAY BRADBURY

SCOTTY

When I was eleven years old, I decided that I wanted to learn ventriloquism.

To this day, I have absolutely no idea where the idea of ventriloquism came from. My class was given a project for a school fair: pick a new skill, learn it, and present it however you choose.

While other kids were off learning to skateboard and all the cool tricks that went with it, I was off to the library to read books and check out videos of creepy dolls that look like they'll come to life while you're asleep and kill you. The kids learning to skateboard were coming into school each day with scabbed-up knees and bandaged wrists. They were learning by attempting to skateboard, falling off, getting a Popsicle from Mom, and getting back on that board. *They were learning by doing.* I, on the other hand, was spending hours upon hours reading, researching, and picking out clothes for the $500 doll I'd somehow convinced my parents was absolutely-necessary-for-this-project-and-I-swear-on-my-life-I'll-use-from-now-until-college-if-you-buy-it-for-me. I read about ventriloquism techniques, watched videos of famous ventriloquists, and flipped through catalogue after catalogue of ventriloquist dolls. I lived and breathed all things ventriloquism.

Except that I wasn't actually *practicing* ventriloquism.

After a month of intense research, the big school fair arrived. Nervous as hell at the thought of performing, but more nervous about the repercussion from my parents if I didn't, considering they'd just invested $500 in what I'd told them was my future career, I turned the presentation over to Scotty, my ventriloquist doll.

It turns out that I did not, in fact, know how to do ventriloquism.

The next hour's worth of visitors were treated to Scotty—who, by the way, looked eerily like the male version of me—greeting them with, "Hey! Hello! How ya doing?!" in a voice that not only sounded 100 percent like my own but was also clearly coming from my moving lips, not Scotty's poorly maneuvered puppet triggers.

Fun fact: if you want to learn ventriloquism, you have to—wait for this plot twist—*practice ventriloquism.*

I'm not telling you this story to give you nightmares about serial killer ventriloquist dolls (though my dad not only still has Scotty but keeps him on a shelf near the front door, nearly giving visitors a heart attack), but to demonstrate a key factor into why most people over-plan and underperform when it comes to creating a new life of health and fitness: *paralysis by analysis.*

PARALYSIS BY ANALYSIS

Most people start backward.

First comes the planning. *Oh, the planning.*

Detailed, down-to-the-minute timelines of each day that include specific times to eat, exact foods for every meal and snack, when to drink water and take bathroom breaks, and a set-in-stone workout routine with a carved-out gym time for each day. They make binders upon binders of workouts, detailing what body part to train on what day, what exercises to do for that body part, and how many reps of each exercise they must do each day. There are shopping lists longer than your average drug store receipt of what to stock up on this week, and a massive fridge overhaul that includes throwing out anything and everything not listed on said shopping list. They spend weeks, maybe even months, getting themselves mentally prepared for this major lifestyle shift they're about to take.

On paper, it's perfect. Now all they have to do is follow the plan and everything will be great, *right?*

If you're not already laughing at the thought of following that plan perfectly, then indulge me.

Make a mental list of all the days in your life that you can remember going 100 percent according to plan. If you're like me, you know your number by the time you're finished reading that sentence because it's zero.

There are two issues with this exhaustive planning. The first isn't the planning itself; it's the *not starting.*

What I learned from my short-lived ventriloquism days is that there's nothing wrong with research and planning. In fact, it's a great tool to utilize. But that's exactly what it is: *a tool*. It's not how the change actually happens.

It's in the *doing* that we make progress.

Had I actually been, you know, *practicing ventriloquism* as I was doing my research, that story might have ended with a contract for Scotty and me to perform weekly standup at the Apollo. *Might*. But because all I did was get my tools ready, without actually utilizing the new information I was learning, I didn't learn or improve.

Most people get so caught up on the planning part of their health and fitness journey that all they actually succeed in doing is postponing the most important part: *putting the plan to use.*

Planning is great if it helps you, but it's the *doing* where you see results.

The second issue with this perfectly laid out roadmap of workouts, meals, and bathroom breaks is the expectation that following such a detailed plan is realistic.

We've now built the event, a major lifestyle overhaul, into *such* a huge ordeal through all this planning that, when it doesn't go according to said perfectly laid out plan, which it won't, we quit.

We're setting ourselves up for failure with unrealistic expectations.

As you embark on your new, healthy lifestyle, there will be days where you have every intention of getting a workout in, and then life happens. There will be days where you meal prep a beautiful, nutritious lunch, and then donuts happen. You will have major successes, and you will hit roadblocks. You will have days you feel unstoppable, and days you feel like complete shit. When you approach this new journey from the standpoint of *Here's my perfectly laid out plan, now I just need to stick to it 100 percent and not deviate*, you're setting yourself up for failure.

Every single time you've attempted to diet in a way that's not sustainable, you've unintentionally reaffirmed some limiting bullshit beliefs. The thoughts of, *See?! Who was I kidding, thinking I could ever change?* or *This stuff just doesn't work for me.* And every time you reaffirm those limiting beliefs, you are literally wiring your brain to experience feelings and take actions aligned with those negative thoughts. And on and on the cycle goes.

If we want to break this vicious cycle, we begin by *taking immediate action.*

Not perfect action.

Not all-or-nothing action.

Not total life overhaul action.

Just one step.

Then another.

Then another.

We take that first step, you guessed it, *immediately.*

One of my favorite expressions in life comes from Ray Bradbury, who advised: "Jump off the cliff and build your wings on the way down." Whether it's starting a business, saying yes to that new job you're not fully qualified for, or dedicating yourself to a healthier life, you don't have to know everything yet.

You'll learn.

You'll adjust.

You'll improve.

First, you need to start.

WHY IT'S NEVER STUCK

If you've started and stopped more diets than you can count and are currently in a place where you're unhappy with your health, you need a new method. As the old saying goes, "If you do what you've always done, you'll get what you've always gotten." Embrace the fact that if you continue to use the methods you've used in the past, you will continue to wind up in the same place.

It's time for a change.

A change *doesn't* mean a new diet. The "old method" wasn't one particular diet or another, it was the whole idea of jumping from fad diet to fad diet.

Real, lasting change comes from getting educated.

Whether it's learning tennis, negotiating like a boss, knowing how muscle growth truly works, or understanding the truth behind nutrition, *getting educated* is always the key to sustainable change.

Anytime you blindly follow instructions without understanding the *why* or *how* behind them, you're limiting the sustainability of the knowledge you're acquiring. You might see results temporarily, but you're doomed to fall right back into your old ways the moment you're left to make the journey alone.

Education is the key to empowerment.

So, congratulations! The fact that you're reading this book right now means you've taken the first step to getting educated. That's massive.

This journey into understanding how health and fitness truly work, not according to fad marketing but according to math and science, will be a continuous one, as is everything in life. That doesn't mean we wait to know it all before we start. It means we take each and every actionable step presented in this book and keep going no matter what.

At the end of each chapter, you'll find a section called Put in the Work. I suggest using a dedicated journal for these sections so you can go back and track your progress. Like everything in life, this section comes down to choice. You get to choose whether you skim through the work or commit to putting aside the two to twenty minutes to take action and make a change. You already know the outcome of skimming over; it's the same life you've been living up until now. I know the results you'll see by taking the time to do the work. It's my hope that you'll find out as well.

As you get more advanced with fitness and nutrition, you'll organically take your knowledge to the next level and up your game. That's how life works: we start where we are, we improve, we learn more, we adjust, we level up.

The same will be true with your health and fitness journey, just as it was for mine.

RACHEL-THE-NEWBIE

I was a complete mess when I started going to the gym. Seriously, I had no idea what I was doing. I sincerely wish I had videos of those days so I could demonstrate to what level that statement is true. I have no doubt some of that old footage would now be a viral gym meme. I used to go to this total meathead gym, the kind where people go with one goal and one goal only: to lift heavy shit. No selfies, no talking, just grunting and massive *BANG*s from weights being dropped. To say I was intimidated is like saying Gandhi was a "pretty nice dude." Accurate, though a wild, wild understatement.

I went to this meathead gym with my good friend, Alex. She'd been lifting for years and was not only much more knowledgeable than I was, but she was also significantly stronger, which frustrated me endlessly.

A typical gym session would go like this:

Alex would go first. I'd walk around her from all angles and take pictures like a total creeper. I'd then do my set, making notes on any form cues Alex gave me. When it came to Alex's second set, I would no longer take pictures or even pay attention to her. I was then too busy referring back to those pictures and searching the internet with my best description of the exercise we just did.

A search for "bicep high cables" would lead me to pictures of fitness models demonstrating the exercise, along with the real name, "overhead cable bicep curls." I would then search "overhead cable bicep curls" so I could bookmark a video of how to do each exercise, demonstrated by a pro.

This process was tedious, and, honestly, a bit ridiculous in retrospect. There are *way* easier methods to learn what to do in the gym. In fact, I've made an entire career out of teaching people how to avoid learning the way I did. But the point is this: I was a mess when I started. I had zero idea what I was doing, took the long route, and made massive amounts of mistakes.

But I started.

And I kept going.

And I kept learning.

By doing.

But that's not the end of this Rachel-the-Newbie tale. We haven't even touched on the worst part: *my nutrition.*

At the time, I was a pseudovegetarian. Pseudo because, while I didn't eat meat on a daily basis, traveling is one of my biggest passions in life, and I couldn't travel to Greece and not try anything and everything on the menu, including pasta with lamb ragù that literally made me cry tears of joy. To be clear, you can definitely build muscle while being a vegetarian or vegan. As you'll learn in this book, protein is protein. As long as you're getting enough complete protein as a vegetarian, you're good to go. But I wasn't. So, I would put all this time and energy into going to the gym, lifting heavy things up and down, taking pictures of Alex, researching and learning, yet barely see results.

You can imagine my level of frustration.

It took me almost a full year to hit my breaking point and finally seek out a coach. When I did, it changed the path of my health and fitness journey for life. What my coach *didn't* do was tell me what to eat and what not to eat. Instead, he taught me the truth about how nutrition works *according to math and science*. He taught me *how* to make choices aligned with my goals and *why* those foods were better choices on a daily basis. He showed me *how* to allow for foods I love that are less aligned and *why* restriction will never be sustainable. He gave me the tools I needed to do this on my own and to understand how it works so I didn't need him, or anyone else, to make it a sustainable lifestyle. He gave me an *education* in nutrition. I then took that baseline education and continued to study, grow, and develop.

While I logically know this wasn't the case, my memory thinks back on that time like Popeye downing a can of spinach.

The results were dramatic. My muscles grew, resulting in not only a healthier body but also heavier lifting in the gym. My energy shot up tenfold, every teacher's dream come true. And that yearly flu most teachers get? It had nothin' on my immune system of steel.

After a year of putting in the work and not seeing the reward, I quickly saw that nutrition was the missing element. Once I understood how it worked, I practiced until it became a part of my lifestyle.

I continued to learn. I continued to tweak. And, most of all, I continued to be *consistent*. That's what matters. As you'll learn in this book, you don't have to make a major life overhaul all at once. You only have to start with small changes and let momentum play its role. *But you must start and keep going.* Get this idea of perfection out of your head. This isn't about being perfect, never eating "bad" foods, or never missing a workout. It's about starting, messing up, adjusting, learning, and, no matter what, continuing.

TRAIN YOUR MIND AND THE REST WILL FOLLOW

Growing up, my brother Jason and I both played baseball competitively. We spent countless weekends at batting cages and going out to the ballfield to play catch for hours on end.

Our dad, David Freiman, had a favorite saying when it came to both baseball and life: "You touch, you catch," meaning if you can get your glove on the ball, there's no reason you can't complete the play. Translation: *we don't half-ass in this family.* If you commit to something (you touch), you do it 100 percent (you catch).

This Freiman mindset did wonders for my work ethic. From the age of twelve on, I had the drive of a Wall Street bigwig and the focus of a college student half a bottle of Adderall in. It also built some pretty set-in-stone beliefs of who I am:

I am the person who gets shit done.

I am the person who knows what she wants and goes after it.

I am the person who is in control, doesn't flounder when making decisions, always has a plan, commits, and executes.

Then, when I was thirty years old, I realized I'm gay.

"Realized" seems like an odd word to most people. Typically coming out late in life means you've been living your life as some kind of emotional ninja called Master Suppressor.

That wasn't the case for me.

Because I grew up with the Freiman mindset of all in or all out, pun totally intended, it never occurred to me that the "weird" feeling I got around some girls was actually what is commonly known as a crush. As you might imagine, this was a major life plot twist. There I was, thirty years old and thinking I knew exactly where I was going with my life, plowing full steam ahead, only to suddenly be punched in the face by this massive realization that I've been living a life that's not fulfilling and not who I really am. It was, to put it mildly, nuclear.

Suddenly, I was the person floundering.

Who am I?

How did I not realize this until now?

I'm the person who knows who she is, knows what she wants, and has a clear path. This wasn't part of the plan!

My concerns had nothing to do with the gay part itself; that made *total* sense to me once it clicked. *It was the beliefs about who I had decided I was and years of stories I'd told myself that were now being rocked.*

It was the only time in my entire life that I didn't trust myself, and it was earth-shaking. In my typical Freiman manner, I went out to "solve" the problem. For months, I thought and thought about how I could learn to trust myself again. I read books about change. I repeated mantras. I worked tirelessly to force trust back into myself. Yet all it did was make me feel worse.

What I was actually doing in my efforts to solve the trust issue was reaffirming the belief that it wasn't OK for me to feel unsettled. I was telling my mind that this was a problem to be solved, not a new life to settle into. I was fighting against myself instead of training my mind to help me settle into this new, empowered, true version of me.

In the middle of this mindset war against myself, I started going to yoga five to six times a week. I don't believe in coincidences, so when I was waiting outside the studio after arriving early for a class one day and my dear friend Tracy, whom I hadn't seen in over a year, walked up, I knew it was for a reason, though I had no idea the impact that moment would have on my life journey ahead. Tracy innocently asked how I was doing. The poor girl had no idea of the floodgates she was about to rip open.

My whole story came rushing out: the distrust in myself, my world feeling shaken and shattered, the fear, the confusion. I verbally vomited all over her and, in true Tracy style, she took it like a champ. After giving me a big hug and taking a few deep breaths together, Tracy calmly and lovingly told me to, and I quote, "Leave it the fuck alone."

She told me to stop trying to force things. To live the life that makes me happy and tell that little voice in my head to shut the hell up when it tried to convince me we were "wasting time" by not solving the issue immediately. She told me to let this unfold organically, and to enjoy the ride.

I will never forget feeling utterly shocked by her advice. *Leave*

*it alone?! That's not the Freiman way! We look for solutions! We fix
things! We don't "let them settle." We settle them, damn it!*

But I took her advice, continued doing what felt right, and, just
as she said, allowed my new life to settle in and become my new
normal with time. Every single time that little voice in my head
spoke up to remind me how out of control I felt, how I didn't know
who I was anymore, how this "wasn't me," I reminded it that it
might not feel like me yet, but we were getting there. I told it that
it didn't need to solve any problem for me, but just take the ride
with me. I spent a tremendous amount of time internally talking
to that little voice. Telling her things like:

I know this feels crazy. It's new, and that's OK.

I know we're not used to feeling unsettled. This is temporary. Just breathe.

*This is scary. It doesn't feel like the life I'm used to. And it doesn't need
to right now.*

*Just keep breathing. Just keep putting one foot in front of the other. Just
keep going, and I promise, we'll come out of it a happier, healthier person.*

That voice had a lot of strong opinions about what I should and
shouldn't be doing. But I just kept reassuring her that this would
take time and we were doing our best. I put my trust in Tracy's
words, and in myself, that I'd come out on the other end a happier, more fulfilled person, and I just needed to trust the process.

And that's exactly what happened.

With time, patience, and continuous training of my mindset, my
"new life" not only became my new normal, but it also became the

happiest, most fulfilled version of my life I have ever known. It no longer seems scary and unsettled. It feels empowered, badass, and exactly where I am meant to be.

Here's what I've learned from both my own experience and my years of work with clients going through major changes in their health and fitness lifestyle: *any change will become your new normal with time.*

The key is, we need to *train our mind* to serve us along the way.

When we go through any major life change, whether it's coming out or getting our health in check, our mind will do everything in its power to convince us as to why it's "not us." You'll soon understand why this is from a biological standpoint and how to change the role of your thoughts.

For now, understand this: if it feels uncomfortable, if it feels like it's "not you," it's a safe bet that it's working. If it felt like the same ol', same ol', well, we already know where that leads.

We're here for new. We're here for change that lasts. We're here for a you that's living the life you deserve.

To get all that, we need to do three things:

1. Get educated. We need to understand *how* and *why* this works so you're set up with the tools you need and are empowered to do it on your own, for the rest of your kick-ass life.
2. Train our mindset along with our body, ensuring our new habits are solidified and we have thoughts that are pulling us toward our goals, not pushing us away from them.
3. Start.

And that's exactly where we'll begin our work together.

Put in the Work

Start. (You can flip the page now.)

CHAPTER II

THE BLUE GORILLA IN THE ROOM: RESTRICTION

"...if you judge a fish by its ability to climb a tree, it will spend its whole life believing it is stupid."
—ALBERT EINSTEIN

YOUR REBEL BRAIN

Let's play a game.

Right now, think about anything *except* a blue gorilla. Whatever you do, *do not* think about a giant blue gorilla. Especially one that's balanced on a little hot pink rubber ball. Seriously. Hippo? No problem. Giraffe? Go for it. But eliminate any and all thoughts of a giant, fuzzy, blue gorilla with its big ol' feet balanced on a tiny hot pink rubber ball, all while holding a miniature-sized banana in his oversized blue gorilla paws.

How'd that work out for you?

Back when I was a teacher, those twelve-year-old middle school kids got a bad rap for wanting to do what they're told not to:

"Lucas, I *just* told you not to play your trumpet out of turn!"

"Halle, why must you insist on taking your phone out in class when you know it's against school policy?"

"James, this is literally the third time in one class period that I've asked you to stop putting your finger in Bradley's nose. Seriously, it's weird dude."

It's easy to blame it on their youth, but, really, this shit lasts *long* beyond puberty. Whether it's picturing blue gorillas or cutting out entire food groups, your mind wants to do whatever you tell it not to. Throughout this book, we'll talk in-depth about the most common weight loss programs on the market, from point systems and frozen meals to eliminating all carbs or staying on a low-fat diet. We'll talk about why some work, why many don't, and, most importantly, how weight loss is something you can 100 percent do on your own without relying on any company or cutting out entire food groups.

Before we get into the logistics of all that, we need to fully digest (pun totally intended) the underlying theme of most diets out there. Most weight loss "solutions" are based on the idea of "Eat this. Don't eat this." In other words, *they're based upon restriction*.

So, let me be clear on this:

Restriction. Doesn't. Work.

If you've spent the past ten years bouncing from restriction-based diet to restriction-based diet and beating yourself up every time you "didn't have the willpower" to stick with it, now's the time to take a deep breath, give yourself an apology hug for all those harsh words you thought each time you caved and gave into temptation, and understand this:

1. As living creatures, we are designed to avoid pain and seek pleasure. Restriction is a form of discomfort. Discomfort is a form of pain. Therefore, *attempting to diet on the basis of restriction goes against our nature.* Read that last sentence again. It's a biggie.
2. Willpower is a limited source.
3. Because of reasons 1 and 2, prolonged restriction leads to our old friend Bingeing.

As we dive into these three reasons, keep this general rule of thumb in mind:

If your current way of eating, or new Diet of the Month, isn't something you can envision doing for the rest of your life, it's time to find a new way of doing things.

JEDI MASTERS, FREUD, AND CARBS

Think about this for a moment:

> What's your knee-jerk reaction when you have an itch? What do you do when you realize you're sitting on your keys and they're creating a bigger pain in your ass than the traffic jam you're currently stuck in?

Unless you're a Jedi Master or Navy Seal, I'm assuming the answer is you make a move to alleviate the situation. Why? Along with making smokers second-guess their oral fixation, Freud, the renowned founder of psychoanalysis, introduced us to something called the Pleasure Principle. In it, he states that there is a basic human tendency to *avoid pain and seek pleasure.* Our bodies have a need to let go of or reduce any tension, pain, or discomfort, internal or external.

In other words, *our bodies don't do well with discomfort.*

They're constantly trying to get back to homeostasis, our natural, comfortable, resting point. Unless you are consciously focusing all your attention on not scratching that itch, you're going to go to town on that itchy son of a bitch. Unless you've Jedi-mastered your mind to not care about keys puncturing your ass, the most logical reaction is to move them. *Quickly.* Left up to its own devices, your body wants to feel good. With or without your conscious effort, it's going to move you away from pain and toward pleasure.

Every. Single. Time.

While itches and key punctures are physical pain, restriction is also a form of pain. More specifically, discomfort. Your body doesn't want to stay in a place of discomfort, so, consciously or subconsciously, it will work to get you out of said discomfort.

Here's the problem: As mentioned, most diets out there are based upon restriction. The entire basis of their program is telling you what you are *not allowed* to eat.

Hour 1: *Today's the day I start my low-carb diet! No matter what happens today, no carbs for me!*

Hour 2: *So far, so good! Yes, I was a bit uncomfortable watching every-*

one eat bagels at the meeting this morning, but I planned ahead with my boiled eggs and I'm good to go! No carbs, here we go!

Hour 4: *Um, wow. People eat a lot more carbs than I realized. I feel like I'm constantly surrounded by bread. And pasta. And donuts. And everything delicious. I mean, ahem, everything carb-based. There are other delicious foods that aren't carbs. *Nervous laugh* Not to worry! I won't cave! Carb-free for me!*

Hour 8: *This is ridiculous! Doesn't everyone in my office know I've cut out carbs?! How dare they stuff their faces with donuts right in front of me!! I WILL NOT EAT CARBS! DO YOU HEAR ME?! I WON'T CAVE!*

Hour 12: *Sobbing* *Must...not...eat...carbs...*

...and that's only Day One.

Or there are the countless programs that tell you the only foods you're *allowed* to eat. Which is a glass-half-full way of telling you that all other foods are off-limits, restricted.

"Yes, hi, I'd like to order the omelet. Egg whites only. Spinach is OK but absolutely no onions. And if it comes with fruit, please don't put it on my plate. Fruit contains sugar, which I absolutely can't have. My trainer has told me that fruit is the devil and the reason I'm overweight. CANTALOUPE KILLS! NO FRUIT! Oh, bacon? Yes, two servings, please."

And, finally, the programs that *only* allow you to eat their specific meals. *Everything else* that doesn't contain their company's label is off-limits:

"Oh, Linda, I'd *love* to go skiing in Tahoe this weekend! The problem is, the only supermarket within an hour of the cabin doesn't carry my frozen meals, so I wouldn't be able to eat for the entire weekend. Bummer. Looks like I'll have to sit this one out."

Which of these methods seems sustainable to you? My money's on *none*.

Telling yourself you can't have certain foods, following a list of "approved" and "not approved" items, or living off of someone else's frozen meals is not only completely unnecessary, but it's also not going to last. Repeatedly telling our body what it *can't* have, whether it's carbs, pizza, or any food missing a specific company's label, creates pressure. We're keeping our body in a state of discomfort, telling it *no, no, no,* without offering another solution, a release where it has options and choices to say *yes* to.

In psychology, this is called *reactance,*[1] when a person feels that someone or something is taking away their choices or limiting their options. As humans, we don't like that. We want to be in control. We want options. We want *freedom,* not restriction.

Every single diet you've tried that was based on "don't do this" was a restriction. As your body searched for homeostasis, its resting comfort zone, you repeatedly worked *against its nature* to resist pain, in this case discomfort.

Without an explanation of why, or, even worse, without a replacement of what to do instead, you were destined to either cave or be miserable, or both.

You were 100 percent reliant on willpower to make it work. And, as we're about to see, willpower is a limited resource.

COOKIE EATERS VS. RADISH EATERS

Have you ever gone into one of the *real* Krispy Kreme stores? Not the pop in and grab a box off the shelf ones. The *real* ones. The ones with the conveyor belt in the middle, so you can see and smell (*oh, the smell*) fresh glazed donuts freely circling their way out of the glorious donut-making machine and onto that magical land called the sample plate?

Imagine I sat you down in the middle of that store, freshly baked donut smell in the air, people happily chowing down on glazed donuts all around you.

I don't think the word *nirvana* is too bold to use here.

Instead of handing you a donut, however, I decide to be a real jerk and give you a bowl of celery. The rule is, you're allowed to eat celery to your heart's content, but under no circumstances are you to eat a donut. What a jackass, I know. After I decide you've been tortured enough, I put a puzzle in front of you. Because we've already determined that I'm a raging asshole, the puzzle is unsolvable, but you don't know that.

Here's the crazy part. Well, second crazy part. I'm fairly certain that insisting you eat celery instead of Krispy Kremes is the first sign of a sociopath. Science has proven that you'd give up on that puzzle *twice as fast* as you would have had I let you partake in those delicious, delicious donuts. Why?

Because donuts make us smarter. Duh.

Also, because this was proven in a study done in 1998 by psychologist Roy Baumeister using radishes and cookies,[2] which aren't as fun as Krispy Kremes, so clearly I had to edit. In this less-exciting-but-probably-more-scientific study, participants were divided into two groups: the Cookie Eaters and the Radish Eaters.

After indulging in freshly baked cookies or munching their hopes and dreams away on radishes while they resisted said cookies, they were given an unsolvable puzzle. Those who'd had to use willpower to resist the cookies gave up on the puzzle twice as fast as those who had been allowed to give in to their craving. What does this show?

Like donuts, cookies make us smarter!

And, willpower is a limited resource.

This is huge for us!

No wonder it didn't last every time we tried to push through a restrictive diet using willpower alone! It's is an exhaustible resource!

If you've spent six months telling yourself *No, no, no!* and depleting your personal level of willpower, well, we've seen how that ends. Namely one more trip on the Self-Fulfilling-Prophecy Bus of *I'll never be able to do this.* If your modus operandi thus far has *been Don't eat carbs. Must...not...eat...carbs...* you're playing for the Radish Eaters, my friend. And, in the real world, your next test of willpower isn't an unsolvable puzzle put in front of you by some dude in a lab coat, it's the birthday cake at your kid's party or the dozen bagels in the staff room.

It's only a matter of time until you throw in the carbs...I mean cards.

HOW TO RUIN YOUR VACATION

Viewing food as "good" or "bad," "allowed" or "off-limits," is a recipe for bingeing.

"But Rachel," I've been told repeatedly, "I can't operate any other way. The second I give myself permission to eat a 'bad' food, I overdo it."

Exactly. Allow me to demonstrate.

A few summers back, my partner, Amanda, and I were visiting her niece and nephew in LA. Because we don't have kids of our own and hadn't yet learned that asking a nine-year-old boy and seven-year-old girl what they want for breakfast will *always* lead you to a donut factory, our hopes for a light vegetarian egg white omelet were overridden by ear-piercing chants of, "Kris-py Kreme! Kris-py Kreme!" In which case the only answer is to reward the terrible behavior in order to make it stop. As is my understanding of how to raise young children.

So, to Krispy Kreme we went. It's important to know that, at this stage of my life, I hadn't had a donut in *five years*. I know. Madness. See, I had spent the last five years "eating clean." Let me be clear: "eating clean" meant eating healthy food *most of the time* until I'd crack and eat a family-sized portion of baked ziti, a large pizza, and garlic rolls all by myself. True story: This was my second date with Amanda. The waitress literally said, "I'm eight months pregnant, and I can't eat that much." Then back to "clean eating" I went.

We have another word for this in the health and fitness world: *bingeing.* It's what happens when you decide there are foods you "can" or "do" eat and foods you "can't" or "don't" eat.

Like donuts. *For five years.*

Anyway, back to our *Adventures in Babysitting.*

This wasn't your run-of-the-mill Krispy Kreme store. This was one of the real ones, as featured in our Cookie Eater versus Radish Eater story, conveyor belt and all. When offered a sample by the employee in his killer Krispy Kreme hat, I smugly responded, "Ew, no thanks. I don't eat donuts."

I can barely write that without laughing at myself now, as the next thirty minutes in that donut shop are now a landmark in my personal history.

The smell of those freshly baked glazed donuts was torturing me. I didn't remember donuts smelling that good. I couldn't help but wonder what I was missing as I watched Amanda and the kids light up with a look that can only be described as pure bliss. Amanda must have seen the look of torture on my face and/or the drool running down my chin and asked if I wanted a bite of her donut.

"*OK,*" I conceded, feeling my willpower break. "I'll just try one little bite."

Do I need to tell you what happened next?

1. I went to the counter and ordered a glazed donut of my own. And a chocolate one. You know, just to compare.
2. Amanda's niece didn't want her second donut. I got up to throw it out for her. And ate it standing in front of the trash can. I'm not proud.
3. I ordered another glazed donut for the road. And by another, I mean another three.

In total, I ate six donuts in a fifteen-minute time span and had a stomachache that spanned the course of five days (i.e., the rest of our vacation) as my five-year-donut-free stomach tried to process, literally, what just happened. Because I had viewed donuts as something "I don't eat," the moment I gave myself "permission," I went overboard. My mind and body went from zero to a hundred *really quick*. The floodgates were open, and boy-oh-boy did I make up for years of lost donut-eating time.

If your relationship with food has been one of "good" or "bad," "allowed" or "not allowed" for the past ten or thirty years, it's no wonder that's the only way you know how to operate! But what if I had learned five years ago that I *absolutely can* eat the occasional donut while still losing fat and accomplishing my fitness goals? That trip to the donut store would have been just another cool selfie I took in a Krispy Kreme hat, as opposed to the day I ruined our California trip with a bellyache that lasted five full days.

When we learn to eat for our goals the majority of the time *while still allowing* for the foods we love that aren't as aligned with those goals, we create balance and, by extension, sustainability. Yet when I tell people that they can lose fat while eating the occasional donut, they look at me like I just told them I was impregnated by a chocolate glazed.

But it's the absolute truth.

Defining ourselves by what we do or don't eat, deciding which foods are allowed and which are off-limits, creating tension and discomfort by trying to diet based on restriction—all of these are recipes for both caving and bingeing because they go against our human nature. And every time we've caved and binged, we've taken our self-defined "failure" as a reflection on our self-worth.

TAKING IT PERSONALLY

As we dive deep into our personal bullshit stories and beliefs, we'll understand not only how we cemented these beliefs but also how we've been stuck on the Self-Fulfilling Prophecy Bus. More importantly, we'll learn how to get the fuck off.

You spent six months telling yourself, *Don't eat the carbs* and the moment (surprise, surprise) that you caved, you took it personally, labeling it as further proof that you're incapable of hitting your goals. I don't care if you've tried five diets or five thousand. If the plan is to continue trying to do this in a way that goes against your human nature to feel good, it will not last. And every time it doesn't last, you deepen those bullshit stories that you can't do this.

I'm here to tell you that you can.

Look, I'm a huge fan of personal responsibility. I'm not here to tell you to point fingers and blame others for the fact that you're not happy with your current level of health. What I want you to understand is that *there's nothing wrong with you.* What's wrong is the *method* with which you've been going about this. And that part's not your fault. There are athletes, professors, and scientists who fall for clever health and fitness marketing every day! Marketing is a sneaky son of a bitch! It wants to keep you coming back, which means keeping you reliant on their product and only giving you as much information as you need to follow that particular system.

It's time for a new system.

Not a new point system, frozen meal program, or food-group-eliminating diet, but a new relationship with health and fitness that's in line with how we are designed, body and mind.

One that's about having options, not doing this based on restriction. One that doesn't require relying on willpower. One that's based on *education* and *understanding how this works*, not blindly following someone's point system with no idea why it does or doesn't work.

As we learn the truth about how fat loss works, not according to mass marketing but according to math and science, as we learn how to shift our mindset to a method that's *in tune* with our nature, not fighting against it, *that's* when this becomes a sustainable lifestyle.

So, think about that blue gorilla if you want to, but throw some trees in there with him. Maybe a kangaroo on a tricycle. Instead of telling your mind what *not* to think about, we're here to learn to give it options.

Like that little hot pink rubber ball, this is all about balance.

Put in the Work

Grab your journal and draw three columns. In the first column, make a list of every single diet you've tried and failed. Yes, it will be a harsh dose of reality to see that list pile up. That's OK. We need to shine the light of awareness on our past so we can learn and move forward.

In the second column, put a brief explanation of how the diet worked logistically. This can be as in-depth or simple as you choose to make it. If you know how it was *supposed to work*, write it down. If you only know *how it was supposed to be followed*, not how it actually worked, write that down.

Finally, using your new understanding of why dieting based on restriction and willpower goes against our nature, write down *why this diet didn't work* in the third column.

Remember, this isn't about making excuses. We're looking for the pattern of restriction that may be woven throughout every past attempt. Once we identify this pattern, we can see why we didn't actually "fail" every single diet on the list. The only thing we "failed" at was trying to use restriction and willpower twenty different times.

Example:

DIET	LOGISTICS	WHY IT DIDN'T WORK
Pete's Point System	Eat only pre-packaged snacks by Pete. I don't know why; those were the only instructions.	This diet was based on restriction. I couldn't eat anything not approved by Pete's Points.
Frank's Frozen Meals	Eat only frozen meals by Frank, two meals a day, then a "free meal" between 500–600 calories for dinner. I don't know why; those were the only instructions.	This diet was based on restriction. I only got one meal a day of choice; the rest had to be approved by Frank.
Low Carb	Eat no more than 50 grams of carbs a day. I think the idea was for my body to burn fat instead of carbs, which was supposed to make me lose fat.	This diet was based on restriction. I spent most of my day thinking about not eating carbs.

Now, make a list of the interwoven themes of your diets. In our example, it's:

- Restriction
- Not understanding *why* or *how* they worked, only what to do
- Limited food choices

Knowing what you know now about human tendencies and willpower, it's no surprise they didn't work. Just think of all the unnecessary blame you put on your past self and the limiting beliefs that blame has led to!

It's time to start letting them go.

Here's your final step: write a letter to your past self, apologizing for the harsh words, the stories your perceived failure led to, and the blame you placed on yourself for trying to force something that went against your nature. This can be a powerful tool for release and a huge step into your new, empowered future when you take the time to do it. Here's a sample apology letter from my client Carly:

Dear Carly,

I owe you a huge apology.

This whole time, I thought you were weak. I thought you had no willpower. I thought you were just not cut out for this weight loss stuff.

After digging deep, what I found was that this has nothing to do with you and everything to do with the way in which I was going about the process.

I was trying to force you to live a life of restriction, which goes against our nature. I was trying to get you to blindly follow someone's system, then expected you to know how to do it indefinitely, without ever learning how!

It seems so silly now, the unrealistic expectations I was putting on you.

And yet that's not the worst of it.

When you "failed," I personalized it. It was no longer just "failing at a diet" but "me being a failure."

It wasn't just "running out of willpower to not eat certain foods" but "me having no willpower."

And those stories have stuck around and solidified for a long time.

I get it now. It wasn't you. It was the system. And we're done with this.

So, I'm sorry. I release all the old pressure, the old bullshit stories, and the old bullshit beliefs those stories led to.

It's time to do this right, once and for all.

All my love,

Carly

CHAPTER III

MINDSET

"Your truth' and the truth' are not the same, even though you have designed your life around the idea that they are."
—GARY BISHOP

I want to let you in on a little secret about me:

I hate cardio.

Run this shit like cardio? No. I run this shit like a person who will do everything in her power to avoid stepping foot on a treadmill.

I know doing more cardio would be good for me. It's great for my heart, it strengthens my lungs, and—let's be honest, this is the real winner—I could eat more calories in a day while hitting my goals. Nonetheless, I still hate cardio.

If Olympic sprinter Usain Bolt were to come up to me and say, "Hey, Rachel! Here's the plan: we're gonna start training you to run a sub-four-minute mile with hopes of getting you into the Olympics!" I'd laugh in his face and run away.

Unfortunately, he's Usain Bolt, so catching up to my slow ass would be easy and the conversation would continue.

In his second attempt, Usain might wise up and say, "Hey, Rachel! Here's the plan: I know you love donuts. What if I could teach you how to burn more calories in a day, making room for more donuts, *and* strengthen your heart so you can potentially live longer, *and* improve your lungs so you can belt out P!nk songs even louder during your workout? Best of all, we'll start with only fifteen minutes per day, five days a week!"

Well, now Usain and I have something to talk about besides what my signature move should be, which is clearly conversation topic number one.

What was the difference in Usain's two approaches?

1. He didn't try to make me do a major life overhaul. Olympics? That's an all-in lifestyle, and one that I have zero interest in living. A sub-four-minute mile not only sounds like a tremendous amount of work, but it sounds like a tremendous amount of work that I am not committed to. But fifteen minutes a day, five days a week? That's not a life overhaul. That's baby steps. Even my cardio-hating ass can handle that.
2. He appealed to my why, the thing or things that light me up and inspire me to work hard. I know, I know. Cheesy fitness buzzword alert. Bear with me—we're not just throwing clichés around, we're tapping into your inspiration. I don't give a shit about running a sub-four-minute mile. I do, however, give lots of shits about eating donuts. A plan that allows me to eat more calories while hitting my goals *and* improving my capacity to entertain the gym with my rendition of "So What" by P!nk? Well played, Usain.

In addition to his mad running and posing skills, Usain understood a key factor to making a lifestyle change. See, there's a reason you've started and stopped more times than you'd like to admit. It's not the slow metabolism your family swears you have or the big hips every woman on your mother's side claims to have been born with.

It's because we haven't *trained our minds* along with our bodies.

We're trying to make outward changes without addressing the internal bullshit that's holding us back. In doing so, we're attempting to start a new life that our old self isn't ready for. This internal bullshit comes in a few forms, all of which we'll dive into together in this chapter:

- All in/all out mindset. This is far and away the number one stumbling block that's responsible for people never hitting their goals. Thankfully, it's a simple fix. Let me be clear: Simple means it's not complicated. Simple doesn't mean easy. It will take constant practice and reminding. It will take identifying and rewriting old beliefs. It will mean going against what you've done hundreds of times before. All of which we will do together.
- Doing a major life overhaul. Trying to go from zero to a billion. Deciding that everything you were doing before was "wrong" and now you're going to "do it right," overnight.
- Relying on motivation. Motivation is bullshit. Period.
- Repeating patterns based on limiting beliefs. Your mind is a tricky son of a bitch. It's wired to win. But if you don't identify what it's winning at, you'll keep running on that hamster wheel of your current life.

All four of these common roadblocks can be eliminated with small changes, time, and practice. When you shift your mindset from *all in/all out* to *always in*, when you learn to view your goals as a "get to" instead of a "have to," when you let momentum play its role, when you identify and rewrite limiting beliefs, you finally understand how to do this as a lifestyle instead of yet another failed crash diet.

Let's start with the single most important mindset shift you can make.

ALL IN/ALL OUT

Sound familiar? You're either on your diet 100 percent or you're eating an entire Meat Lover's pizza in one sitting. You're either in the gym five days a week or you're glued to your couch yelling at the art teacher with a $3 million budget on yet another unrealistic home decor reality show, "You can change the color of the paint on the freaking walls!!"

The biggest roadblock for most people has little to do with the logistics of health and fitness. It's this all in/all out mindset.

This mindset, my friends, is complete and utter ridiculousness. Why? Let's take it back to my middle school band teaching days for a moment.

Imagine that your eleven-year-old daughter, Katie, decides to play the trumpet in the school band. If you're anything like my parents, the first thing you do is buy ear plugs and designate a practice area outside.

Katie's band teacher has advised the new students to commit

themselves to practicing just fifteen minutes a day, five days a week. Eager and excited about the new dying cow noises she's producing on her instrument, Katie races home from school on Monday and proceeds to entertain the neighbors with fifteen uninterrupted minutes of what sounds like the family cat being stepped on repeatedly. Fun times. Tuesday rolls around and the performance is repeated. But HOLY SHIT THERE'S SOCCER PRACTICE ON WEDNESDAY! Call the band director and THE coast guard BECAUSE OBVIOUSLY little KATIE has to give up her dreams of BECOMING a professional musician. Miss a day of practice?! CLEARLY, she can't go on!!!

Um, ridiculous, right?

The obvious answer for Katie is that one day of missed practice means *zero* in the scheme of her entire life of music ahead of her. Plus, the band director said five days a week, which means she has Thursday through Sunday to make up for the day. And even if she didn't, the world isn't ending. She'll get back on her schedule next week.

So why do we do this to ourselves when it comes to health and fitness?

There's a beautiful meme someone once sent me that shows a determined woman jogging through a beautiful, serene forest and eloquently states:

"If you're tired of starting over, keep going."

Someone get that author a Hallmark contract. Here's my version:

"Stop. Fucking. Stopping."

Seriously.

Somewhere along the line, someone, probably a women's health magazine, decided to sell this idea of "all in/all out." I'm either on my diet or eating tacos like they're the base of the food pyramid. I'm either in the gym five days a week or I'm seeing exactly how long it will take for me to physically meld into an extension of a couch cushion.

Care to know the secret to doing this successfully?

Go grab a highlighter. Or some ink to tattoo this to your forehead.

I'll wait.

Here we go:

KEEP GOING.

Seriously.

Eat something not aligned with your goals?

Enjoy it. Then get right back on. Not on Monday. Not next month. The next freakin' bite.

Miss a workout because of, I don't know, *life*?

Good. Enjoy the rest day. Get back on. Not next Monday. Not next month. Tomorrow.

Going to your child's wedding and want to enjoy the freakin' $1,500 cake YOU PAID FOR, GODDAMN IT?

Eat the freakin' cake and stop thinking about calories at your child's wedding! Then get back on with your goals. Immediately.

Traveling to Belize for your twenty-year anniversary and only able to use the resort gym three of the seven days you're there?

You're in fucking Belize! Put this book down, stop thinking about the gym on the four days you don't have access to it, and enjoy your vacation! Then get back on your routine when you're home.

Get out of this mindset of all in/all out.

You're in.

You'll mess up.

You won't be perfect.

But you will be successful if you keep going.

This concept is simple. That doesn't mean it's easy. Most of us have spent our entire lives thus far living all in or all out without ever questioning if there's another approach. Here's the good news:

You just have to decide.

Today.

Right now.

And every time you catch yourself saying, *Well, I already ate one slice of pizza, may as well finish the pie* or *I already missed two days at the gym this week, may as well give up on my twelve-week challenge,* rewrite the story:

> HOT DAMN, *that pizza was delicious! Glad that craving's out of my system. Now right back to eating for my goals!*

> Or, *Man, I missed the gym on those two days I was away! Time to get right back to it and keep building those habits!*

It's a simple shift. It's also the most powerful one you can make.

So, make it.

Right now.

You're in.

THE MAJOR LIFE OVERHAUL VS. MOMENTUM

One of the funnier conversations I overheard during my middle school teaching career, tied with the time I heard an eleven-year-old girl telling her bestie that she broke up with her boyfriend because she "just didn't see it going anywhere," was the following:

> Thirteen-year-old girl: "I can't wait for our pizza party tonight!"

> Bestie: "I thought you decided to become a vegan this morning?"

> Thirteen-year-old girl: "I did. It's my cheat day."

Clearly the dramatic life change of the past six hours was more than her poor thirteen-year-old heart could handle.

But this is what we do, isn't it? We decide it's time for a change, and boy, oh boy, do we make one.

Enter the Major Life Overhaul:

The epic fridge clean out.

The grilled chicken and brown rice.

The veggies. Oh, the veggies.

Aaaaaand...the inevitable binge.

The *I've been so good, I deserve...*

The *I've been craving chocolate for two weeks, so I'll just have a bite... or an entire bag.*

The *I'M ONLY HUMAN! HOW DO YOU EXPECT ME TO LIVE A LIFE WITHOUT CHEESE?! STOP THE INSANITY!!!*

I'll be blunt here: if you're currently eating Mickey D's five times a week and your plan is to switch to a life of chicken and rice, you're setting yourself up for failure. Hell, if being healthy meant only eating chicken and rice, Arnold Fuckin' Schwarzenegger would be setting himself up for failure. This is not about perfect. This is not about restriction. Go reread chapter II if you need a refresher. And this is certainly not about a major life overhaul.

When you try to do this as a massive life overhaul, you create pressure. And anytime you create pressure, you create stress. And anytime you create pressure and stress, you turn the sit-

uation into a "have to." And anytime a situation turns into a "have to," you won't stick with it long-term.

I don't care if you're talking about eating healthy, running, ballet, or going to work with calendar-level-cute puppies, the moment you *have* to do it, the moment you create pressure, you will lose the excitement, burn out, and quit.

Do me a favor before we continue: Take three seconds and put two fingers lightly on the inside of your wrist. Feel a pulse? Good. Then this applies to you. Read on:

You don't have to force this.

Because our body naturally wants to feel good and is always searching for ways to avoid pain and seek pleasure, we can start with simple swaps. When we trade soda for water or have grilled chicken instead of fried, our body goes, *Holy shit, that feels good.* **What else can I do?**

So maybe the next day, you swap out a soda for water, opt for a plant-based dinner instead of your usual steak, *and* go for a fifteen-minute walk. And your body goes, *Holy shit, that feels good.* **What else can I do?**

When we let momentum play its role, we're accomplishing two things:

1. **We take the overwhelm away.** Our goals become achievable because we're not focused on some far-off, massive end result. We're simply focused on one doable step at a time.
2. **We keep it exciting.** By starting with small changes, we

keep our minds and bodies engaged, continuously looking for more ways to feel good.

Little trumpet-playing Katie's parents didn't hand her a trumpet, sign her up for private lessons, and schedule her audition for the New York Philharmonic all on the same day. She started slowly. Fifteen minutes a day, five days a week. One day, Katie's parents might go to her band director and say, "Katie went from practicing fifteen minutes a day to thirty. She really seems to like it and is getting better. Where can we go from here to help her improve?"

It happened organically.

She started *slowly*.

She put in *consistent* work.

And when she progressed, they looked into next steps.

This is how to make health and fitness a sustainable lifestyle.

Stop with the unsustainable Major Life Overhauls.

Stop with the all in/all out way of thinking.

Start.

Right now.

Today.

This minute.

As we talk in detail about the truth behind how fitness and nutrition work, you'll have a plethora of actionable steps you can take for your personal health and fitness journey. Make sure you take them. For example, in the Put in the Work section in this chapter, we're going to write down three *small* changes you can commit to *today*. The great part is, you don't need to wait until you finish this book to begin. You just start.

"But Rachel, I don't know where to start!"

Remember, we're not overhauling here. I have every confidence that you can common sense your way into three actionable steps. Let's practice. Choose the option that you believe will be a healthier first step:

Fried chicken or grilled chicken

Soda or water

Elevator or stairs

One Krispy Kreme or five (zero is not an option in my book)

See? Baby steps. But here's the key: *You gotta do 'em.* Reading about it, thinking about it, actively imagining yourself doing it won't cut it. The more you do it, the easier it gets. Remember, our bodies want to feel good. Choosing just one off the list above will leave your body wanting more.

So, start with one.

MOTIVATION VS. YOUR WHY

Now that we're done with this starting and stopping bullshit and we're starting with small steps and letting momentum play its role, we can start to dig a little deeper into what makes you tick.

Let's say you're not currently in a consistent gym routine, and I call you and ask you to meet me at 4:00 a.m. for a workout. We both know how that story ends: either with you hanging up on me or calling me a slew of names I've only been called one other time in my life when I accidentally cut someone off on the highway and they threw a half full soda can through my open car window while spewing a stream of obscenities like I've never heard.

In other words, it's a no from you.

If, however, I tell you, "Meet me in the gym tomorrow at 4:00 a.m. I have a bag with $100,000 in cash for you," chances are you'd show up. Or call the cops. Or both.

Nothing changed logistically between the two scenarios. It's the same ungodly time of day. It's the same drive to the gym for you. The only thing that changed was your *why*. Your reason. The pull that got you to do something you're not used to doing.

Before we get too into this *why* stuff, I want to be clear on something: I do not believe in relying on motivation. Motivation is fleeting. It's like a Tinder date: fun when it shows up, but typically unreliable and likely to leave you disappointed in the long run.

While I'm a huge fan of reading motivational books, listening to motivational podcasts, and watching motivational videos to *fuel* the fire, they themselves are *not* the fire. Your *why* is the fire and your *habits* (we're getting to those) keep the flame alive. Motivation is that extra pump of lighter fluid you pour on now and then so you can beat your chest and do your best "I am woman, hear me roar!" chant. It's not sustainable. It's not reliable. And if you spend your days waiting to feel motivated to take the steps necessary to reach your goals, you won't. Nobody who has ever accomplished any goal in life did so by only putting in the work when they felt motivated. Motivation is not the answer.

You need to be crystal clear on *why* this is a *must* for you. I'm not saying *must* lightly here. If this is a "Meh, lemme give this a go," we both know how that story ends.

When you decide this is happening *now*, no matter what, well, *that's* the pull from your *why*. Then the key is to keep it. There will be days when you mess up. There will be days you're busy. There will be days you simply don't feel like it, also known as lack of motivation. Those are the days when your habits will see you through, *if your why is at the forefront of your mind* to keep you going.

Here's a brief list of common *why*s I've come across as a coach:

- My doc says I'm going to die young if I don't get my health in check
- I feel like shit all day, every day
- I've avoided mirrors for over ten years
- My four-year-old asked me if I'm pregnant (and I'm not)
- I'm tired of being tired all the time
- I want to eat more donuts in a day (OK, only one person has said this)

Your *why* is personal. It could be as serious as a heart attack or as fun as wanting to add more calories in your diet. Whether it's serious or fun enough for you to stick with it is up to you. The point is, there's a reason you're reading this book and a reason you've decided that you *must* make a change.

That's your why.

Motivation is a little push. Your *why* is a pull. It's what gets you out of bed in the mornings when it's still dark out. It's the reason you get to the gym on the long days when Ben and Jerry are calling your name from the couch.

It's the reason this is a *must* and not a *should*.

Identifying your *why* and continuously keeping it at the forefront are crucial, especially during the beginning stages of building new habits. A simple way to start figuring this out is to simply complete this sentence:

"I *must* do this right now because [insert reason]."

No filtering. No excuses. One hundred percent brutal honesty.

That's your *why*.

Got it? Make sure you write it down because we're not done.

At this point we know:

- We're in it to win it. Never again with this starting and stopping bullshit.
- We're starting with small steps and letting momentum play its role.
- If we're relying on motivation, we won't hit our goals. Our *why* is what will keep us going.

The good news is, your *why* is powerful shit. The reality, however, is that if it were *that* powerful, you wouldn't be reading this book. Knowing why you must do this is an important stepping-stone to keep you on track. But to make a lasting lifestyle change, we need to dig deeper.

We need to figure out *why your why hasn't been enough to get you to stick with it.*

Which leads us to the final step in this mindset work.

To fully understand and, more importantly, break through what's held you back in the past, we have to dig into something uncomfortable, something you've unwittingly worked your whole life to cover up.

We must call ourselves out on our own bullshit.

SHAME VS. EMPOWERMENT: MY WHY

Back in those beginning gym days with Alex, I didn't talk to anyone else too much about my newfound hobby of weightlifting. It was up there with incessant partying and sowing some serious wild oats: just part of what I did in a day and not serious enough to warrant a full-fledged convo.

Then, about six months into my training, I was talking to one of my best friends about a mutual friend who had recently done their first bodybuilding competition. Without a second thought, my dear friend said, "I seriously cannot think of a more selfish way to go through life. Can you imagine caring about every single calorie you eat and constantly looking at yourself in the mirror like that? It's disgusting."

Well. You can fill in the rest from there: Shame. Embarrassment. Feelings of selfishness.

I had never thought about it that way. To me, lifting just felt good. I loved the challenge. I loved the mental focus it took. I loved pushing myself past where my mind wanted to tell me my physical limits existed.

But...I guess she had a point. There *is* something selfish about caring about how you look and feel...*isn't there*? Suddenly, my love of the sport felt shameful.

I never posted a single selfie on social media in that entire first year of training. I mean, how much more self-obsessed could you get?! When my family eventually started asking about the time I was spending in the gym, I tried my best to gloss over the subject. The seed had been planted by someone I love and respect that this way of life was selfish, and I had accepted it as truth.

Let's pause here to point out that *I was an adult* at this stage in my life. Thankfully, because I was thirty and not three, I was able to eventually take a step back and do some self-reflection. After a full year of hiding my shameful little self-obsessed secret, I finally took a breath and asked myself, *Why **am** I doing this?* Was it only to get a glimpse of a bicep bump in the mirror? Was it really to look good naked? Or was that statement just one person's outside perception of another human being, whose *why* they had zero idea about?

When I was able to identify my *why*, it not only helped me release the bullshit selfish story I was carrying around, but something bigger also happened:

It empowered me.

I realized that my *why* is *because of how I feel.*

When I lift, I feel strong, fulfilled, confident—the best version of myself. And when I show up as the best version of myself, I can then help those around me feel all those positive attributes for themselves as well. It became clear that it's actually the *least* selfish way I can live my life.

But imagine if that comment was made in front of me when I was a young child, in those early years when our brains are sponges at picking up new information and storing it as fact, unquestioned. Even worse, imagine if it was made *repeatedly* when I was too young to step back and process.

This, my friend, is where the majority of our bullshit beliefs began.

Maybe it was hearing your mom and your aunt repeatedly talk about "that skinny bitch" at the nail salon. Translation to a child: *We don't like women who are skinny.*

Maybe it was hearing your dad and grandpa telling everyone who would listen that life's too short to not eat the cake. Translation to a child: *If you want to enjoy life, don't have boundaries.*

Wherever it comes from, that mother is planted deep and *every single time* something happened in your life since then—a skinny person was rude to you, a fit person rejected the cake at your birthday party—that belief went deeper and deeper.

These belief systems are at the root of why you've never experienced lasting change. *They* are the reason you've made progress, and, at the first hiccup, or cupcake, you've decided, *Who am I kidding, thinking I can change? This is who I am.*

You are self-sabotaging because your new life doesn't fit in with your old belief system.

Read that again. That's not a cop-out. That's not an excuse to fall back on and do nothing.

That's a starting point from which to move forward.

LIMITING BELIEFS AND $10,000 IN KRISPY KREMES

There's a reason that so many lottery winners blow all their newly found cash within the first five years of their big win. Yeah, it's partly because seeing how many donuts $10,000 will buy you sounds *freaking amazing*, but it's mostly because said lottery winner is still the same person inside.

If they didn't build the habit of a monthly budget when they had $100 in their bank account, adding a bunch of zeros didn't do anything but give them more money to blow through without a second thought. If they were stuck in a cycle of getting money and then immediately spending it because deep down they believe money is the root of all evil, all this newfound cash did is give them a larger sum to get rid of ASAP. If they struggled in a life of poverty because they hold a subconscious belief that they're undeserving of money or being rich makes them a greedy, selfish person, it's pretty clear that getting back to their comfort zone of being a nongreedy poor person is of the utmost importance.

Their habits, their mindset, and their belief system haven't caught up to their new way of life. Until they do, their new way of life isn't sticking around very long.

This, my life-lottery-winning-because-you're-reading-this-book friend, is true of your past attempts to live a healthier lifestyle. You could lose 150 pounds, get all the plastic surgery a doc will allow you to get, and look smokin' hot to everyone around you, but if you still tell yourself you're a lazy piece of shit every day, guess how you're going to feel? I can write out daily workouts for you, give you step-by-step meal planning guides, and teach you self-empowering mantras to scream buck naked in front of the bathroom mirror, but if you still believe that you're undeserving of looking and feeling good, or deep down you believe that looking and feeling good makes you selfish, or that it's going against your family, or that your family will see you as a "skinny bitch," it won't last.

Life is *all* in our mind. That's not some hippie voodoo stuff. That's neuroscience, my friend. As we talk more about habits, you'll start to see just why this stuff is so important. You'll understand that all this limiting belief bullshit is actually *wiring your brain* to bring you back to your old life. You're trying to run a marathon with your foot glued to the starting block. It's time to recognize it and let go.

Trying to change your body without training your mind is a vicious cycle, one that most of us have experienced countless times up until now. You make some changes, see some results, and then you get dragged right back to where you started, reinforcing the limiting belief that you can't do this. And on and on the cycle goes.

Train your body. Train your mind. *That's the key to making this a sustainable lifestyle.*

Before you go shelving this book right next to *101 Mantras That Never Worked*, let me be clear on something: I can sit in front of a mirror all day long and sing motivational songs to my biceps encouraging them to *grow, baby, grow*, but unless I get my ass into a gym, ain't nothin' happening. The same is true of your mind. If you don't train it, if you don't put in the work each and every day, nothing will change. You'll be right back to hangin' out at Mickey D's with the dude who just spent the last of his $10 million on the dollar menu.

The good news? This stuff is life changing. No, more than life changing: life *unleashing*. When you train your body *and* your mind, you become a fucking powerhouse. A force to be reckoned with. The best version of yourself that you never even knew was possible.

Before we dive into *actionable* tools to train your mind, start by locking this belief into place:

Just like that lottery winner, if you do not first call yourself out on your bullshit, identify those deep-rooted limiting beliefs, and start to self-identify with this new, healthy you, you *will* self-sabotage your way back to your comfort zone. You *will* find yourself back where you started, reaffirming the idea that this "just isn't for you."

This *is* for you.

This is for *everyone*.

The logistics of health and fitness are math and science. And you, magical as you are, do not defy the laws of math and science. What's held you back isn't some freak gene that's blocked the science of fat loss to work for you. It was your mindset.

If we want to change our current situation, it begins with training our mind.

Put in the Work

Write out this declaration in your journal.

"Today [date], I am in.

No more stopping and starting.

If I eat something not aligned with my goals, I get right back on.

If I <GASP> miss a workout, I get right back to it.

Not next week. Not next month. Right away.

[Sign]"

Below it, list three things you commit to doing *today*. Then answer these questions.

- Why am I committed to doing these? Why now?
- How will I continuously remind myself of my *why*, including the days when I simply don't feel like putting in the work?
- When I try to picture myself with the body, energy, and health of my dreams, what are the immediate thoughts that rush in? No filtering. No editing. Let the bullshit pour out.
- Now that you've got a few out, let it flow. What other bullshit are you telling yourself? Are you afraid of what someone will say? How you'll be treated? Believe you don't have the time? Fear of failure? Shame if you start and stop again? (You've already signed on that you won't, don't forget.) Get it all out.

CHAPTER IV

THOUGHTS-FEELINGS-ACTIONS-RESULTS

Think of it this way: the input remains the same, so the output has to remain the same. How, then, can you ever create anything new?
—JOE DISPENZA

THE KEY TO HAPPINESS

I know you thought you were reading this book solely to learn about health and fitness, but, *bonus!* I'm about to lay the secret to happiness on you.

There's a very real pattern that exists in your life and taking control of it is the key to not only making change that lasts, but also to unlocking every dream, every goal, and every aspiration that you hold. The pattern goes like this:

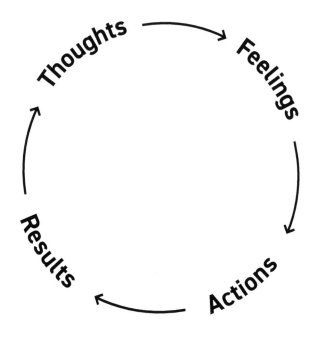

The thoughts we think lead to the feelings we experience. Those feelings we experience lead to the actions we take, which lead to the results we see in our lives. Those results lead back to the thoughts we think. And on and on the cycle goes.

The key is this cycle exists whether we're consciously choosing those thoughts, feelings, actions, and results or not. And, more often than not, we're reacting to circumstance rather than choosing how we want to think, feel, and act. By shining the light of awareness on our thoughts, we can take control of the cycle.

This starts by understanding that all meaning, to every circumstance in life, is self-made.

SPLASH MOUNTAIN AND OTHER TORTURE DEVICES

Nothing in life has any meaning except what we give it. And the meaning we give the situation determines the thoughts we think and, therefore, the feelings we have about it. Nothing more clearly demonstrates how true this is than a roller coaster.

I have never met a human being more afraid of roller coasters than my mom. There's a memory etched in my brain from the time I was nine years old and we took our first family trip to Disney World. I made the dreadful mistake of sitting next to my mom on Splash Mountain, a water ride consisting of two drops: the medium-sized warm-up and the big ol' main attraction drop. It should be noted that I was nine and well within the ride's age and height limit, so that big ol' main drop wasn't actually *that* big. Nonetheless, I will never forget the approach of the drop. I could hear my mom frantically repeating something between a prayer and a slew of words I wasn't yet allowed to say. As the moment of doom approached, her inappropriate prayer turned to absolute silence as she braced for what she believed to be certain death. We began the descent, that moment where you can only see empty space in front of you, and she grabbed the nearest thing available to hold onto: me. The force with which she squeezed my hand was, in retrospect, impressive but, at the time, shocking.

After what seemed like two days later, but, in reality, was more like five seconds, my mom released my hand, took a deep, calming breath, and sighed, "Thank goodness that's over."

"Mom," I replied, "that was the warm-up drop."

Roller coasters are the perfect example of how our thoughts affect our feelings. I love roller coasters. As I approach the pinnacle before the drop, I'm filled with feelings of excitement, eagerness, anticipation, and thrill. My mom's feelings, on the other hand, are of panic, anxiety, despair, and regret for being there in the first place. I'm sure thoughts of payback for making her get on the damn thing would also creep in at some point.

We're both on the same ride. We're both in the same moment in time. It's clearly not the actual event that's causing such different emotions to the same stimulus. So, what's responsible for the drastically different states of my thrill versus my mom's complete panic?

Our thoughts.

As our roller coaster rounds the top, giving a clear view of what the next five seconds of our life entails, my interpretation—the thoughts I'm having about the meaning of that moment—is the polar opposite of that of my mom.

Because I interpret this event as thrilling, my thoughts are along the lines of:

Oh man! This is gonna be awesome!

My belly is flipping, and I love it! This rush is incredible!

The second I get off this ride, I'm going right back on! I could do this all day!

Because my mom is fairly certain this is how she leaves this world, her thoughts are more along the lines of:

I'm going to die. Right here, right now.

Who the hell gets on a machine designed to plummet you toward the ground this fast?!

Get me off this thing. GET. ME. OFF. THIS. THING. I'm gonna die. I'm gonna die. I'm gonna die!

The place and situation are the same. It is *only* our interpretation of the event and, therefore, our thoughts about the situation, that differ. This applies to *everything*, from roller coasters to your relationship with exercise to your feelings about your physical appearance. It's our *thoughts* that determine what we experience. And those thoughts are 100 percent responsible for what comes next: *our feelings*.

Why is this so important? As we're about to see, the way we feel determines the actions we take in this world, and the results we experience. Those actions and results become our daily habits. That alone is a huge deal, yet it's just the tip of the iceberg. As we'll discuss in chapter V, "Habits," *a whopping 95 percent of the time, our mind is run by our subconscious brain, acting on autopilot.*[3] Think about what that means:

Left unchecked, our Thoughts → Feelings cycle isn't a result of conscious thought, but of automatic response. We're running on autopilot the vast majority of the time yet expecting different results to come about in our lives.

To quote one of my favorites from the '90s, we need to check ourselves before we wreck ourselves.

FEELING OUR THOUGHTS ON AUTOPILOT

While you are a unique, sparkly unicorn, we're often surprised to find out just how many of our feelings in a day aren't the result of free will or our individuality but, rather, this automatic response.

When I had my initial thought on top of that roller coaster of, *Oh man! This is gonna be awesome!* my body physically reacted in particular ways: my heart started beating faster, my adrenaline was pumpin' hard-core, my palms felt sweaty, and my stomach felt like I must have swallowed a mouthful of butterflies on the roller coaster's ascent, which would really be a nightmare, given my irrational fear of butterflies. I didn't have to think about the chemical reactions happening in my body. Its automatic response was to set off that chain of events based on my thoughts and beliefs about my current situation. I had trained my mind to associate roller coasters with excitement, so my body physically responded to that trigger in a preset way.

My mom's body, interestingly enough, had nearly the exact same physical reaction. Her repeated thought that death was surely lurking on the other side of that drop led to a bodily response of a rapidly beating heart, adrenaline galore, sweaty palms, and metaphorical butterflies in her stomach—in this case, the biological response to *fear*. She didn't instruct her body to react this way. The mere thought and belief that she was going to die triggered a series of internal events that her body is conditioned to act out.

So, if we were on the same roller coaster *and* showing the same physical reactions, why, when asked to describe the event, would it sound like I just took the joyride of my life while my mom took a trip on a torture machine? Because of our interpretations of the event, our body's innate physical response was triggered without our conscious thought. We had an experience, we determined what that experience meant to us, it produced a feeling, and our body produced a physical reaction to that experience.

It all started with our thoughts. The rest was autopilot.

Throughout our lives, our bodies have been conditioned about how to respond to particular thoughts. Some of it is biological. The sweaty palms, racing heart, and spiked adrenaline that my mom experienced were not unique to her, but how most bodies respond to fear. The sheer state of panic she slid into, however, is a trained response. My mom has trained her body to go into full-out panic mode when it encounters a situation where she believes her life is at risk.

Compare this to, say, your best friend, Zoey, who worked for the Peace Corps and backpacked through the Amazon forest solo prior to having kids and taking them to Disney World. Having faced major life risks well beyond that of Splash Mountain, her reaction might be slightly different. While a flash of fear may enter her mind, Zoey has trained herself to deal with dangerous situations well beyond this one. She takes a deep breath, acknowledges the fearful thought, reminds herself of the security checks and inspections all roller coasters must go through, and reframes the situation as one of excitement instead of fear. Within seconds, her hands are in the air, and she's *woohooing* with the best of them. Zoey has trained her mind to evaluate her thoughts and, in turn, she can control the corresponding feeling that results.

While we may not be able to stop every thought that flashes through our brain, we can learn to acknowledge the thought, pause, breathe, and reframe our interpretation into one that better serves our goals, just as Zoey did.

Let's be clear that this is not about *suppression.* There is value in simply acknowledging thoughts and letting them pass, as well as valuable information to be found in evaluating certain recurring thoughts and understanding what led to them. *Why* do you dread the gym? *What belief* is leading you to think people are staring and judging? We can learn a tremendous amount about our limiting beliefs by acknowledging these recurring thoughts and understanding where they originate. The goal, however, is not to *cling* to every thought that goes by or interpret it as Truth.

It's about which thoughts we choose to give our attention to. In meditation, the analogy of a mountain is often used. You are the mountain, watching the clouds (thoughts) go by. You're not attached to them; you are simply observing their passing. From this space, you can then do the work to reframe the situation and focus on new, empowering thoughts that better serve your goals. In doing so, you can choose the feelings you feel and the actions you take.

Doing so also breaks the repetitive thought loop we may not even know is going on internally.

50,000 THOUGHTS ON REPEAT

If you were to step back and listen to that little voice running in your head all day, you would be shocked to hear how many of your daily thoughts are repetitive:

> *Ugh, these pants feel tight. I can feel them digging into my belly. I need to lose weight.*

> *Seriously, why did I wear these pants today? I knew the second I put them on this morning that they didn't feel comfortable and now I'm stuck in this meeting, distracted by the fact that they're cutting off the circulation in my stomach.*

> *I can't wait to get home and change into my PJs. These pants are the worst. I'm never wearing them again. I think I might have a permanent scar where they're digging into my belly. Stupid pants.*

We have an average of 50,000 thoughts per day.[4] If we're walking around repeating the same thoughts over and over, and we've trained our body, usually unconsciously, to respond to those thoughts with a particular feeling, we're walking around feeling the same feelings the majority of the time!

We're living the same life experience day after day after day.

I'm laying a truth bomb on you right now:

*Until you put in the work to consciously take control of the meaning you're giving to situations and, by response, the feelings your thoughts are producing, you **will** continue living in the same emotional states for the rest of your life.*

When we train our minds to interpret events in ways that serve us, our corresponding feelings will in turn change to ones that empower us.

If your current thoughts about the gym sound like: *Ugh. I hate that place. I feel like everyone's watching me and judging,* how are you going to feel? Tense. Anxious. In a state of dread.

When, however, we train our mind to focus on the good, our feelings follow suit.

Man, I feel strong as hell when I lift. Yeah, the gym can be intimidating, but the more I go, the more comfortable I feel. Let's get another day on the books! How do you feel now? Vivacious. Eager. Lit up.

Same situation. Two very different thoughts. Two drastically different feelings.

Our days turn from *Meh* to *What a freakin' amazing day!*

The events in your day may not have changed. You may still wake up late, scarf down breakfast in your car, go to the same job, leave work late, and have paperwork to do when you get home, but you can *choose* how to interpret these events. Is that breakfast in your car a hassle or is it a good thing your super healthy protein smoothie is not only serving your nutrition goals, but also portable, making it easy for you to drink it without being late to work? Is your job a pain in your ass, or is it the ideal situation, as even getting out late still allows you enough time to squeeze in the gym before going to get the kids and get your paperwork done?

The situation you're in is irrelevant. It's your *thoughts* about the situation, your interpretation of the event, that determine how you will feel in every area of your life.

As we're about to see, when your thoughts and feelings shift, then so do your actions, and, finally, your results. And when we experience positive results, it leads to positive thoughts, which starts our loop all over again:

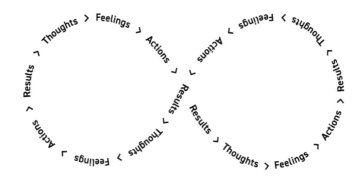

Until we consciously do that work, we're destined to live the same life, the same day, over and over again.

There's an appropriate expression about this: "Wherever you go, there you are."

Many people try to outmaneuver their thoughts, moving to a new state, going on an elaborate vacation, setting a new goal at work, buying a new car, all in a desperate attempt to change things up. The issue is, once the excitement of the new calms down, *there they are*: same thoughts, feelings, actions, and results. While having goals and dreams is a valuable part of human existence, and while vacations and relaxation time are important to hit the refresh button, they are not the answer to a happier, more fulfilled life. If we don't put in the work to train our thoughts and, by extension, our feelings, the results of those goals once attained will leave us back in the exact same place as before.

You can't fix an internal problem with an outside solution.

Let's do an experiment:

Take a moment and try to catch your reflection in something full-length, where you can see a glimpse of your entire body. Without filtering, pay attention to every thought that instantly flashes into your head. Fair warning: you have to be quick to catch these thoughts. We often don't want to admit we're thinking these things, so they flash through just long enough to make us feel crappy, without hanging around long enough to be a conscious thought we're aware of.

What were some of the flashes you caught?

For many people, it's along the lines of:

Ugh. How did I let myself get like this?!

Ew, my nose is too big.

I'm so skinny, it's disgusting.

I'm so fat, it's disgusting.

Look at me. No wonder I'm single.

It's painful to acknowledge, I know. But think about this:

We're walking through our lives, feeling low energy and blah most of the day. Not only are we not sure *why*, but we barely even question it, having accepted it as a result of the current situation in which we live. We're blaming our external circumstances for how we feel inside. Meanwhile, we're having these thoughts, telling ourselves how despicable we are, every single time we catch a glimpse of our reflection! We're telling ourselves, *I'm disgusting*, then wondering why we don't feel happy in a day and expecting a new car or house to change how we feel!

The great news is you can save your cash. You don't need a new house, car, or vacation to start living a life where you feel true, deep happiness; where you feel energized and passionate; and where you feel empowered rather than shrunk down and stuck. The only thing you need is to get your mind healthy, along with your body. This begins by paying attention to the thoughts we're having and the feelings they're producing.

As with everything, from limiting beliefs to nutrition, we must first shine the light of awareness on a situation before we can have real, lasting change.

THROWDOWN IN THE SHOWER

Your thoughts are the most powerful thing you have. They literally determine your future. Why? Because your brain can't tell the difference between what's real and what's a thought in your head.

Remember that monster fight you had with your spouse in the shower? I mean, you weren't *in* the shower having the fight. It was just you, in the shower, mentally *rehearsing* what you *would* say, were the fight to occur. Your spouse was out with friends, none the wiser that this hypothetical argument was in the works.

You list every piece of evidence you have for why you're right, counter every one of your spouse's hypothetical rebuttals, and even envision your Oscar-worthy storm out when your spouse doesn't understand why you're so right in this situation.

By the time your ears are squeaky clean, how do you feel? Chances are you're pissed. Super pissed. Your muscles tense up. Your heart is beating faster. You're breathing heavy. Your face is flushed as blood enters your limbs and extremities to prepare for action. These are all the biological responses to anger.

But, wait. The argument never really happened. This was all in your thoughts. So, why is your body reacting as if your spouse is in that shower, arguing right along with you?

Our brain cannot tell the difference between events that are real and events that we visualize with both thought and emotion.

Had you simply thought, *I think I'll pick a fight with my spouse*, chances are you wouldn't find yourself heated well beyond the water setting in your shower. It was the *emotion* behind those thoughts that triggered a physical response from your body. In your head, you were thinking and feeling just as if the fight was actually happening. Your brain, in response, sent signals to your body that a fight was actually taking place, and your body responded accordingly.

Studies have been done on both musicians and athletes that reveal our brainwaves reflect this truth: our brain responds the same, whether the event is happening or being felt as if it was happening. In one musical study,[5] a group of participants was asked to play a sequence of notes on the piano as their brains were scanned in the region connected to their finger muscles. A second group was asked to only *visualize* themselves practicing the same sequence. A comparison of brain scans showed the brains of both the piano players and the visualizers to have virtually the same wave patterns! In other words, the brain reacted the same way whether they were physically playing the piano or actively visualizing the action.

This is huge when it comes to your health.

If our brain can't tell the difference between an event that actually happened and one that we've imagined with such clarity and emotion, *we can feel the way we want to feel before we've made a single external change in our life.*

This means we can begin to rewrite those repetitive, limiting thoughts into new, empowered ones, whether they're true in this exact moment or not.

Let's look at a few common ones.

I'M TOO WEAK FOR THE GYM.

Say that out loud. How do you feel? In a telling muscle strength test,[6] a participant is asked to hold her arm out while a partner gently pushes down while the participant resists. The second time, the participant is instructed to focus on a negative experience: feelings of shame, embarrassment, weakness, anything blech. When the partner pushes down, it's found that muscle strength often decreases by as much as 50 percent!

Telling yourself over and over that you're too weak to do something is setting yourself up for failure. Putting the science aside, you can feel it in your body just by just thinking the thought. If you're attempting to force yourself into a gym, a yoga class, or a spin class with the repeating thought, *I'm too weak*, you're running on empty before class begins.

What if we change that thought to: *I'm a badass. Watch me rock this.*

Before that little voice in your head starts telling you that you're not actually a badass and you're never stepped foot in a gym so who are you to say that, remember, your brain doesn't know the difference between the thoughts you think with emotion and your current life situation. You're going to be feeding it information anyway, so why not make it an empowering game and feed it the good stuff? Repeat it. Feel it. And walk into that class like the badass you are.

I'M ALWAYS TIRED.

Again, say it out loud. Just reading those words makes my body sink lower in my chair, my shoulders slump, and my energy level drain. Yet most of us walk around with this thought on repeat, telling it to anyone and everyone who will listen. Ask someone at work how they're doing and, more often than not, the go-to response is some variation on how tired they are. What an energy suck.

What if you *decide* that you're the person with crazy amounts of energy? It doesn't matter if it doesn't fully feel that way *yet*. Once you get your health and fitness in check, that part will come. But the first step is to *believe that's who you are*. Say it over and over. Every single time you catch yourself thinking about being tired, remind yourself, *I am the person with crazy amounts of energy*.

I CAN'T DO THIS.

Back when I was a middle school teacher, the number one rule in my classroom was that the word *can't* was banned. I would explain to my students that this wasn't rainbows and unicorns "You can do it!" stuff; this was neuroscience. When you think the thought *I can't*, you're telling your brain and, by extension, your body, that this is not possible. It responds by shutting down, no longer searching for the *how*, because, according to what you just told it, there is no *how*!

If, however, you make a simple shift from *I can't* to *How can I?* that creates a very different feeling. Now we're looking for answers instead of shutting down.

Embarking on a healthy lifestyle takes time, practice, and being gentle with yourself. You'll have days you totally rock it and days you give in to more donuts than you'd like to admit. You'll have weeks you're hitting personal records in the gym and weeks you miss days you didn't intend to. Telling yourself *I can't do this* every time there's a setback is sending your brain and your body the message that you're defeated. Asking *How can I make a better choice next time?* or *How can I prepare in advance for this situation next week?* puts you in a place to search for answers. It puts you in control of the situation instead of falling victim to circumstance. Most of all, it leaves you feeling empowered that you can and will do this.

It all begins with your thoughts. Choose to give your attention to thoughts that serve you. When that little voice in your head tells you it's not true, remind it that your brain doesn't know the difference, and repeat the new, empowered thought over and over until you accept it as truth.

Feel the feelings that follow.

Live in that space.

Own that shit.

THOUGHTS DETECTIVE, FEELINGS DOCTOR

As we've seen, *every single thing* that you feel throughout the day is a result of your thoughts. This means we can work backward.

Begin with the habit of checking in with your feelings and using them as a signal to check in with your thoughts. A great way to do this is by keeping a small notebook with you throughout the day, or start a note in your phone designated solely for check-ins. As you go about your day, be conscious of moments where you sense your feelings shift. You can also set an alarm in your phone to go off a few times a day as a reminder to check in with how you're feeling and where your thoughts are at that moment.

- You suddenly have a wave of excitement. Pause. Check in

with your thoughts. What had just flashed through your mind? Write it down.

- You have a pit in your stomach that wasn't there two minutes ago. Freeze. Check in with your thoughts. What's going on up there? Write it down.
- You wake up feeling anxious. Don't move. Check in with your thoughts. What's on your mind? Write it down.

The point isn't to judge any thoughts. We're not trying to convince ourselves not to have these thoughts. Remember, you are the mountain watching your thoughts go by. Our goal with checking in is to start to identify patterns.

Are there recurring thoughts that lead to recurring feelings?

Do you constantly find yourself thinking about how you've tried every fad diet in the book and nothing's going to work, leading to that stomach pit? Write it down.

Is the thought of going to the gym causing you anxiety and fear? Make a note.

Do you feel anger and resentment when you see someone fit eating junk food? Note any repetition you see as you go.

This process takes twenty seconds to do. It doesn't matter where you are or what you're in the middle of doing. Give yourself the gift of that time to pause, check in, and jot down your results.

As we're about to see, our actions and results come from these thoughts and feelings. If we want to change our physical world, we must first pause and identify what's going on internally.

ACTING FROM OUR FEELINGS

The reason it's so important to get control of which thoughts we give our attention to and, by extension, the feelings we experience, is because our feelings lead to our actions.

If you've ever taught children, led a meeting, come home to other people at the end of a long day, or had a conversation with another human being, you know firsthand how your feelings directly influence your actions, as do the humans with whom you interacted.

Imagine you're a teacher. Ten minutes before the school day starts, an irate parent barges into your classroom to accuse you of picking on her child. Despite the fact that you've personally volunteered to stay after school to tutor this child, this parent is accusing you of singling her out, grading unfairly, and playing favorites with other students in the class. You do your best to keep cool, but, as the accusations fly, you feel yourself trembling with anger and frustration. Eventually, the principal has to be called in to remove the angry parent, mere minutes before your class walks in.

Your thoughts are stuck on the accusations just spewed at you. Your feelings tread a fine line between *What the hell just happened* and fantasies of running into that parent in a UFC ring. What do you think your actions are going to be like that morning? When little Monica comes in and goes directly over to Toby's desk to chat rather than sitting at her own desk and taking out her assignments as she knows she's supposed to each morning, will you take a deep breath and calmly redirect her? Or will you be more likely to snap, releasing some of that anger you're holding from the morning's encounter?

Same scenario, but this time, you arrive in your classroom to find that your spouse had somehow arranged for an early morning delivery. There on your desk are two dozen roses with a note saying, "For my superhero. I'm so proud of you." You feel loved and appreciated. Mere minutes later, your students enter. After the *ooooohs* and *ahhhhs* that undoubtedly follow as the kids see flowers on their teacher's desk, you're all smiles the rest of the day. This time, you pop over to Toby's desk to see what he and Monica are chatting about and even jump in with a couple of jokes before redirecting her back to her seat to get on task.

You're the same person. They're the same kids. But the actions of your morning took two very different turns, all because of your thoughts and, by extension, your feelings. Your thoughts affect your feelings, which affect your actions.

This cycle works in every single area of our lives. As you embark on your health and fitness journey, understanding this cycle is vital to your success.

Let's say part of your plan is to go to the gym for thirty minutes a day, four days a week.

Monday, you crush it. Tuesday, you get it done. Wednesday comes along, however, and you find yourself dreading the gym. All day long, there's this pit in your stomach about the fact that you "have to" go to the gym after this long day of work. You feel *bleh*. You're dragging. It's like a weight is on your shoulders the entire day but you don't have the energy to lift it off.

Pause. Breathe. Without judgment, check in, *backward*.

What action am I avoiding? *I don't want to go to the gym.*

What am I feeling? *Dread. Frustration. Avoidance.*

Where are my thoughts? *I'm supposed to do bicep curls. Last time I did them, I felt weak. It was frustrating. I love training my legs because they're strong. My arms just make me feel bad about myself.*

By tracing our actions, or lack thereof, backward, you've now identified what's *really* going on. You now have the opportunity to make a new choice or reframe. Now that we know the issue isn't with actually going to the gym but frustration with training a certain body part, you can choose to either switch around your workout schedule, saving your arm workout for a day where it feels less daunting and encouraging yourself to get to the gym with the incentive of training a different body part that you enjoy more, or reframe the thought: *I'm surprised to find out how much stronger my legs are than my arms! I bet in a few weeks the increase I see in my arms and upper body strength is going to be massive since I've never focused on training them before. I'm going to keep a notebook so I can watch the change develop! Day One of Operation Build Some Gunzzz begins today!*

Forcing yourself to take new actions will only get you so far. The moment any activity becomes a "have to," you're setting yourself up for burnout. The key, therefore, is not to focus on the action itself but to identify the *feeling* behind the action and the *thought* leading to the feeling.

KUMBAYA, HEMP SEEDS, AND MINDFUL EATING

Working backward from our actions is a powerful tool when it comes to mindful eating as well.

I'm going to pause here and be completely honest: for years, I avoided reading any article or having any conversation that opened with the words *mindful eating*. I naively thought it was some hippie rainbow, unicorn, and fairy dust kind of stuff. I pictured long-haired dudes in sandals sitting around a campfire, singing "Kumbaya" before eating their hemp seeds and goji berries.

What I've found, however, is that mindful eating is an incredible tool for noticing patterns. It's especially useful when it comes to emotional eating and cravings, common struggles many of us face where we turn to food as a comfort, a way to change our emotional state, in times of stress or sadness. Taking the time to identify what's going on in the moment and what's leading to our actions allows us to both make a better choice and prepare for future events.

It's 8:00 p.m. and you're sitting on your couch watching a romantic movie while going over some paperwork. As the lead couple onscreen reaches that fateful moment where they decide if they're going to fight for their relationship or walk away, you realize you've dropped all your papers as you've unconsciously moved to the edge of the couch, grasping onto the cat, tears rolling down your face. Without a second thought, you hit pause, deciding you need some ice cream to get through this climactic scene.

Pause. Breathe.

Action: *Craving ice cream*

Feelings: *Sadness, worry, heartbreak*

Thoughts: *Is she going to be alone? I feel alone. Why can't I meet somebody normal? How many more online dates am I going to have to go on before I meet someone I can cuddle on the couch with at the end of a long day instead of watching sad movies with my cat?*

The point of this exercise isn't to say you should never eat ice cream. If, at the end of that thirty-second check-in, you decide you really want ice cream, eat the ice cream! As we'll learn, when you redefine your relationship with food, there are no "bad foods." The point is that we now understand you're turning to ice cream to comfort your feelings of loneliness. Knowing that, you could choose to turn off the movie and do some journaling, call a friend, switch to a comedy, or call that guy you've been scared to call. You can *choose an action aligned with your goals* because you now understand the thoughts and feelings behind your actions.

Mindful eating can be as simple as taking thirty seconds to think:

What action am I taking right now?

What am I feeling?

What thoughts are leading to this feeling?

It can also include a journal to look for patterns. For example:

DATE	TIME	WHAT I'M DOING	WHAT I'M ABOUT TO DO	WHAT I'M FEELING	WHAT I'M THINKING
9/20/19	8:00 p.m.	Watching Lifetime	Eat ice cream	Loneliness, sadness	I want to meet someone I care about.
9/25/19	8:30 p.m.	Watching *The Bachelor*	Eat cake	Jealousy, isolation	I want to go on a date with someone I connect with.

A few more days of this, and it becomes clear that sweets are your go-to to change your emotional state when you're feeling sad and lonely. By shining the light of awareness on this tendency, you can choose a new action in response to the feeling, prepare for this action by stocking up on healthier sweet options such as fruit the next time you food shop, or choose a new nighttime activity to unwind at the end of the day. Preferably one that doesn't leave you crying with your ol' pals Ben and Jerry.

Whether you're a teacher starting your day, someone starting their new fitness routine, or a single woman watching a romantic movie and using food as comfort, the actions you take in this world produce the *you* that you put forth. You can post motivational memes all day long, but it's your actions that define what you do or don't do in your life.

To start showing up as your best, bravest, most empowered, badassiest self, you must begin by becoming aware of the thoughts you're thinking and the feelings those thoughts lead to. When you learn to identify what's going on internally and make choices to focus on what best serves you, your actions will reflect those empowered choices.

THE RESULTS OF OUR ACTIONS

Our thoughts affect our feelings, which affect our actions. It follows that your actions affect your results. But that's not the end of the cycle. This is a loop. Your results, in turn, affect your thoughts, and on and on the cycle goes.

It is because of this loop that I am such a huge fan of momentum. As discussed in chapter III, people often set themselves up for failure by trying to do a major life overhaul and go all in/all out. Their loop goes something like this:

Thought: *I **have** to change. That's it. No more junk food. Exercise five days a week. Today is the first day of the rest of my life, and I'm 100 percent in.*

Feeling: Excitement mixed with pressure, nervousness, and more pressure

Action: Pushing through feelings of pressure and relying on motivation for this new life to make choices aligned with goals 100 percent of the time

Results: *Ugh, I was spot-on with my goals all week then I not only caved to coffee cake in today's work meeting, but I also have such a bad stomachache from eating it that I have to skip the gym today. It's all messed up now. Who was I to think I could do this? Guess I'll try again next month.*

Compare this to someone whose loop includes small changes, allowing momentum to play its role in the process:

Thought: *It's time for me. I'm going to make my health a priority once and for all. I'll start by swapping out soda for water for two of my three meals today and going for a twenty-minute walk with my partner tonight.*

Feeling: Excitement. Both of those goals are very doable and some quality time in the evening sounds delightful.

Action: Both goals complete!

Result: *I feel amazing! What else can I do tomorrow to keep this feeling going?*

Momentum is oh-so-important because in completing those small, actionable steps, we create a result that *feels good*. It empowers us to want to do more. Our thoughts, in turn, are filled with *Look at me go!* and *Damn, I feel good! I want more of this!* Those thoughts bring about good feelings, which lead to more inspired actions, which bring about results aligned with our goals, which then lead to more good thoughts, and around and around the cycle goes! Before we know it, we've sealed those habits into place and we have ourselves a full-fledged new, healthy, empowered lifestyle.

Watching my client Dana go through this was a beautiful example of the Thoughts-Feelings-Actions-Results loop at play.

When Dana came to me, she felt stuck. She'd struggled to lose the twenty pounds she put on after having her son and felt like she'd tried everything. In our initial conversation, I asked her to envision herself with the energy, body, and health of her dreams and to tell me, unfiltered, what thoughts immediately come to mind. Here was her response:

"It's never going to happen. And even if it does, it won't last. I use food as a crutch. I'm an emotional eater. And if there's one thing I've learned in life, it's that something's always going to happen, and that something will always lead me to ice cream for comfort. I just feel destined to stay at this weight for the rest of my life. Sometimes I think I just need to accept it as a part of getting older. Like, I had my son, now it's his turn to live his best life, and it's time for me to stop worrying about mine."

Ouch.

Yet so many people share these beliefs: *I think I just need to accept it as a part of getting older. It's time for me to stop worrying about my life and focus on my family. I feel destined to stay at this weight.*

What feelings do thoughts like that lead to? That's exactly what Dana and I discussed next. Her answers included: "Stuck," "Frustrated," "Wanting to cry," and "Defeated."

And the actions those feelings lead to? We can guess that one from her initial response: Dana has self-identified as an emotional eater, so she deals with these low-energy feelings by turning to food, namely ice cream.

Her results, therefore, are to stay exactly where she is, and even gain some weight over time.

Her thoughts are leading to feelings of frustration and being stuck, which are leading to actions that are causing the exact result she's frustrated about! And when she doesn't see the scale move due to these results, her thoughts are right back to *See? I knew I was destined to stay in this unhealthy place forever*.

In order for Dana to change her results, we must begin with her thoughts.

Let's talk about the best tool I know to do just that.

TALK TO YOURSELF LIKE A KINDERGARTENER

Imagine for a moment that you're sitting on a park bench, reading this book, lost in thought over how the hell someone goes from being a band nerd to a fitness pro all within one lifetime, when suddenly, a little girl no older than four years old runs up to you, sobbing her little eyes out. You stoop down to her level and calmly ask her what's wrong.

Between sobs she manages to squeak out, "I...*gasp*...can't....*snot bubble*...tie...*more gasping*...my...*more snot*...shoooooeeeesssssss!"

More manic sobbing.

Do you:

1. Immediately start screaming at her, telling her what a loser she is and that she'll never be able to tie her shoes, so she may as well give up now.
2. Console her. Tell her everything's OK. Gently show her how to tie her shoes and allow her to practice, encouraging her to try again and tweak her technique as she makes mistakes.

I'm sincerely hoping that B is the no-brainer answer for you. If not, a job far away from children is highly suggested.

Now, swap out the four-year-old girl for yourself and the shoe tying for your last attempt at a weekly gym routine or a new diet plan. When you tried and failed, how did you speak to yourself internally? Did that little voice in your head talk to you like option A or option B?

For most of us, it's laughable to even imagine being that gentle with ourselves. It would feel silly to talk to ourselves in such a gentle manner. Awkward, even.

Let me ask you this: in which scenario above is the little girl more apt to learn to tie her shoes?

So, *why is the answer any different for you?*

Let me pause here and answer the most common concern I hear at the thought of being gentle with oneself. Right now, that little voice is probably telling you that your toughness on yourself is what gives you your edge. That the second you start being kind or gentle with yourself, you'll become weak. Or lazy. Or unsuccessful.

Sound about right?

So, let's try this:

Take a second and think about your favorite teacher when you were in school. Whether it's been five years or fifty, you know the one. That one. The one that first flashed into your mind. Seriously, stop overthinking this.

How would you describe that teacher?

They may have, and probably did, set the bar high. They may have been strict. A real tight-ass, even. But chances are they were also fair. And encouraging. And made you believe you could do what you set out to do. They set that bar high, but they were also there to help you reach it. They pushed you to grow more than you knew you were capable of, but they did it in a way where you felt empowered, not belittled.

So why do you insist on treating yourself any differently?

If you want to change your results, we must begin by changing your thoughts. I'm about to share with you the single most effective tool I have ever personally used to change my thoughts, the way I speak to myself internally, and, by extension, my feelings, actions, and results. It is literally the number one exercise I know to begin to change your mindset for anything and everything in life. It's also the most ridiculous-feeling exercise I've ever done. And I say that as someone who once tried lifting weights while in a headstand position.

So, ready for the world's most awkward game? The good news is it's all internal. In other words, you'll feel like a dope, but no one will know. The best news is, when you commit to it, it works.

For the next week, commit to talking to yourself like a kindergartner.

Seriously. Like, overdo it.

Thought:

> *Damn it! I told myself I'd go to the gym four days this week. Once again, I'm only going to make it two. I'll never commit to a schedule!*

Pause. Breathe.

Internal convo:

> *Wow, finding four days a week for the gym is a bigger challenge than I expected! This is going to take some planning before the week gets going. You know what, though? I went two days this week, and I loved how I felt after. And, hell, that's two more days than I went last week! That's momentum to keep me going right there! I'm proud of myself for not only getting a couple days in but for recognizing that I need a plan to make this work.*

I know. You're cringing just reading that. Your internal voice is having a field day telling you to just skip this section already because you *know* it's not in you to do something so ridiculous.

It does feel ridiculous...*and it works.*

After a week, a little red flag will automatically start to go up whenever harsh words start in your head. After a month, you won't need to force the convo so much. At some point in the near future, you'll look up and realize that the way you're naturally talking to yourself has done a 180. Suddenly, that little voice is your best friend, the coach that pushes you, and that best teacher you ever had all rolled into one.

Talking to yourself like a kindergartener is the key to unlocking new, empowering thoughts that will, in turn, change your feelings from pressure and frustration to curiosity and excitement. Those new, energized feelings will then lead to actions aligned with your goals, leading to the results you once deemed impossible. Those results fuel the fire of these new, empowered thoughts, and now we're in a very different, much healthier loop.

ELI'S KINDERGARTEN TRANSFORMATION

When I introduce this concept to my clients, I ask them to journal about it in detail.

My client Eli's account of her experience is such a powerful example of why this works:

> "I've been spot-on with macro tracking for a week and a half now. I'm starting to form the habit of inputting all my food into my app. I'm doing better with getting closer to my numbers. Overall, I've been feeling great. For the first time in a long time, I feel like I'm in control of my health and nutrition.
>
> "Today, however, I just caved. I didn't sleep well. I woke up late, tired

and cranky. I grabbed a Pop-Tart as I quite literally ran to my car. A freakin' Pop-Tart! Who eats those anymore?! But that's where my mind was. *Screw it*, I thought, *I deserve a day of whatever I feel like.* I remember that being my exact thought.

"Obviously, I felt way worse after eating the Pop-Tart. Not only was my stomach making weird noises, but my thoughts were also running wild: 'See? No self-control. You always have and always will self-sabotage. You're kidding yourself thinking this time around will be any different.'

"At that point, I thought about doing the talking to myself like a kindergartner technique, but I was still in Screw It All Mode, so I didn't.

"I got to work late, and, as always, someone had left old bagels and donut holes in the meeting room. All week, I had walked by them without a second thought, happily knowing I had brought plenty of food with me to keep me full through the day. Today, however, all bets were off. *Whatever*, I thought, *I already had a Pop-Tart. May as well.*

"Five donut holes later, I was at my desk, fighting back tears. I felt like shit. Physically, mentally, everything. I ran to the bathroom, locked myself in a stall, and cried.

"It was there in the privacy of that bathroom stall that I finally took a few long, deep breaths and had the conversation in my head. I literally pictured myself kneeling down to my four-year-old self and talking to her. Picturing my younger self helped me feel less silly about it, I think."

"OK, Eli, what's going on?"

"I just feel...frustrated. Why do I do this? I'm tired. I'm burned out. I need a break. And then I self-destruct. I eat shit I know I shouldn't.

I think thoughts that don't serve me. It's like I just default to full-out meltdown mode."

"I understand. Anything else?"

"Yeah, I think I'm feeling extra frustrated because I *know* I can do it this time. I mean, I'm doing really well with macros. Not having to restrict my food choices is really helping me be successful, and I know it will work. So why am I doing this?

"I pictured my current self giving my younger self a long hug while we took a few more deep breaths together. Then current Eli spoke to younger Eli in a calm, soothing tone:

"'I'm so proud of you. The fact that you know you can do this is huge. That's the confidence we've been looking for. This is a change, and you're doing your best. Maybe today was a sign to show us that days where we don't get enough sleep will take a little extra preparation to ensure we're still set up for success. We can use how terrible we felt this morning. Let's remember what it felt like and use that as inspiration to make better choices next time. The day's not done. Right now, in this moment, let's take a deep breath, write this off as a valuable lesson, and turn it around. The fact we're having this convo shows *so* much growth. We've got this.'

"I left that bathroom stall feeling like a new human being. Not just from who I was that morning, but from who I've been for the past forty-two years. It was the first time in my life I was kind to myself. And I had never felt more empowered.

"I always thought being gentle with myself would make me weak, unmotivated. What I learned that morning was that I become my most powerful self when I am my best coach."

Put in the Work

Now it's your turn. This exercise requires that you monitor your thoughts and have an internal conversation. Every single time you catch yourself being harsh, pause, breathe, and have an internal conversation the way you would with a four-year-old. Remember, feelings are often the best cue to check in with our thoughts!

You can picture your own child, your niece, nephew, grandchild, a made-up child, or even your four-year-old self, which is often a powerful tool.

Be gentle. In this conversation with a child, there's no need to lie or pretend the event didn't happen. The point is to reframe, to point out the growth and the lesson with which to move forward. Be encouraging, the way you would be with someone you love and want to see succeed. After all, isn't that what we want for ourselves?

Remember, if you feel ridiculous, you're doing it right. You can get that inner voice to calm down by simply acknowledging it. Agree with it that this feels silly, but you're willing to stick with it anyway. If it helps, put the silliness on me. Tell it, *You're right. This feels unnatural and very unlike me. But that Rachel chick seems to know what she's talking about with this stuff, so I'll try this out only because I'm putting my trust in her and we'll see how it goes.*

Grab a journal and make some notes about the experience. As we read in Eli's story, having powerful experiences where we feel a shift can fuel the fire to continue to put in the work.

It is only by first shining the light of awareness on our thoughts and reframing them that we can change how we feel throughout the day. It is through these new, empowered feelings that our actions and, therefore, results will change. And the results we bring about on a daily basis form one of the most vital components of who we are today: our habits.

CHAPTER V

A TRIP TO THE CREEPY FARMHOUSE: HABIT

"We are what we repeatedly do. Excellence, then, is not an act, but a habit."
—ARISTOTLE

This Thoughts → Feelings → Actions → Results stuff is a big deal. It is through this cycle that we are building the most influential factor in our current lives: our habits.

Our current state in every area of our life is a result of our habits.

If we want to change the current state of our lives, we need to begin by taking a hard look at the daily habits we've built, consciously or unconsciously.

Ready? Buckle in. We're about to go somewhere no gym meathead has gone before: *neuroscience*. But in a fun way, I promise.

Imagine you're standing in an overgrown field. At the other end of this field, you can *juuuust* make out a farmhouse that you'd love to check out. Because, you know, who doesn't want to venture into a creepy old farmhouse by themselves? You start dredging your way through the overgrown grass, forcing through the mess despite the shit smacking you in your face, the thorns poking into your legs, the who-knows-what crawling on your arms. Fun times. Eventually, you trudge through that hot ol' mess of a field and arrive at your creepy farmhouse. *Woohoo! Mission accomplished!*

The next day, you find yourself back at your original starting point. You decide you really enjoyed wandering around that farmhouse and want to do it again. Apparently spiderwebs and scary noises do it for you. No judgment. So, you start off on your journey once again. This time, however, you can just barely make out a trace of the path you took yesterday. It's not worn away and enjoyable by any means, but you can at least see where you put a break in the grass and more or less follow the way.

The third time you make this weird , creepy journey, the path is a bit more worn. It gets easier. By the seventh or eighth time (seriously, you need some new hobbies), you have a clear, worn path on your hands. The trip's pretty easy by now. In time, you might decide to make this a real thing. You know, share the creepiness with other people. So, you throw some cement down and seal the path. Now, my friend, you have a full-blown road on your hands.

Plot twist: this process is your brain.

This is how we learn.

And this learning process is why you are at whatever stage you currently are at, in every area of your life.

BUILDIN' HABITS LIKE A BOSS

Our brain creates neural pathways every time we learn something new. Whether it's playing the note C# on the violin, speaking Korean, developing a belief that we're smokin' hot, going to the gym, *not* going to the gym, or telling ourselves we're destined to be overweight, literal wirings are taking place within our brain. With each action and each repeated thought, pathways are being created.

Each time you "walk that path," practice the action, think the thought, do whatever it is that wiring was created to do, this stuff called *myelin* acts as the cement, sealing that connection (pathway) and making the trip easier and easier to take. In fact, our brains are *designed* to clear the path for you, to make it easier to get from point A to point B with repeated time and practice.

It does this through the creation of *habits*.

Since science is always attempting to come up with quirky little sayings to make learning fun, here's an oldie but goody: In 1949, psychologist Donald Hebb introduced us to what's now known as Hebbs Law.[7] In its science-made-fun form, it states that *neurons that fire together, wire together*. In short, when neural impulses are sent on these journeys repeatedly, our brain thinks, *Huh. She's thinking this thought/doing this action a lot nowadays. I better make this easier!* So now *more* neurons join the party, making the message clearer and faster to transmit and, eventually, acting on autopilot.

In other words, it forms a *habit*.

This is great news for three reasons:

1. **Anyone can learn anything.** While some may be genetically predisposed to physical traits that make, say, learning the violin slightly easier, or building a booty that won't quit, any human being can put in focused, deep practice (or, in the latter case, deep squats) and progress. It's simply a matter of repeating correct patterns until the journey on the pathway gets smoother and smoother.

2. **You can choose which pathways you build.** If myelin is coating the neural connection each time we give it focused attention, and if repeated thoughts and actions are causing neurons to fire together and make that path smoother, here's a thought (pun intended), in the most scientific way I can put this: stop giving attention to the shit you don't want to cement. Every time you ruminate on how you've tried to lose weight thirty times and each time resulted in gaining even more, well, you now understand what's happening. You're literally wiring your brain to believe this as your truth. This also means that developing new beliefs is as simple as establishing which thoughts would serve you and focusing on those.

3. **We act according to our beliefs.** The you that exists today is 100 percent a product of the thoughts you think over and over again, and the actions those thoughts bring forth. Those neural connections that have been sealed in tight for the past twenty, thirty, forty, fifty, or sixty years have resulted in the actions you take on a daily basis. And the actions you've taken, or haven't taken, have resulted in the you that's currently reading these words. That's a great thing! You're a badass. You've accomplished a lot in your life. People love you. That's also your roadblock. In any area in your life that you've repeatedly tried to change, only to wind up back where you started, that yo-yo is happening because your brain is wired to believe that its current state is the "correct" one. So, how is that good news? Every single thing you would like to improve in your life

is possible. It's simply a matter of rewiring your brain. Which isn't as painful as it sounds.

Before we dive into these three powerhouses of truth, we need to understand why this stuff is so important. As human beings, free will is kind of a big deal. Many believe it's what makes us who we are. Yet, truth bomb alert, *the majority of what we think and do in a day isn't the result of free will but the result of habit*. To fully understand why, we first need to understand how the human mind works.

Our mind is made up of the conscious mind and the subconscious mind. Your conscious mind is your logic and reasoning. It's in charge of actions and thoughts you're focused on at the moment: You're deciding if you should eat a donut. You're lifting a weight. You're putting the weight down to free up a hand with which to eat more donuts. Your subconscious mind is the involuntary stuff: memories, feelings, beliefs about ourselves. It's the reason you believe you're destined to be fat so you shouldn't eat said donut. It's the story you've accepted as truth that you're weak, so you don't lift the weight.

As we learned in chapter IV, *95 percent of our actions in a day are run by our subconscious mind. Ninety-five percent!*

Think about that: we're running on autopilot, responding to situations the *same exact way, over and over, day in and day out,* according to how our brain has been wired over time through those thoughts, feelings, actions, and results. According to our habits.

We think we're simply deciding (conscious mind) if we want to eat a donut. The reality is that behind the scenes (subconscious mind), there's a whole lot of action going on: limiting beliefs and bullshit stories galore, feelings and responses being triggered by those thoughts, and, ultimately, a decision as to whether to eat the donut or not *that was primarily made by that behind-the-scenes, subconscious action.*

My client Teri saw this clearly after some deep work into her subconscious beliefs. When Teri came to me, she felt like she was always self-sabotaging but didn't understand why.

> "I literally stood there, staring at an apple in my left hand and a chocolate croissant in my right. It was straight up out of a movie where there's the angel on one shoulder and the devil on the other. Logically, I knew I should go for the apple. I'm working to lose weight, and it's clearly the healthier choice. But I could think of nothing but the chocolatey goodness that lived inside that croissant.

> "While I stood there, staring from my left hand to my right like I was watching a ping-pong match, I kept having this flash in my mind. It was me as a kid, sitting at the kitchen counter in my childhood home, watching my parents have breakfast. They were happy and smiling. Drinking coffee and eating, you guessed it, chocolate croissants. This was long before their horrific divorce.

> "I didn't fully understand why this image kept flashing through my mind, but there it was. I finally thought, *Screw it*, threw the apple back in the bin, paid for my croissant, and happily devoured it. I say happily, but that lasted all of the two minutes it took to eat the damn thing that took me twenty minutes to decide on. What followed were feelings of regret, and a massive stomachache.

> "Why do I do that?!"

The image of Teri's happy parents wasn't a coincidence. It was her subconscious mind reminding her that food is a comfort. Chocolate croissants reminded her of a time when her home was peaceful and happy. Food was a central part in this memory. In that moment, Teri's need to feel comforted overrode her logical brain telling her to make a healthy choice. While on the outside, it looked like a test of willpower, Teri was really using her conscious mind (the mind making a simple decision: apple or croissant?) to fight against her subconscious mind, that deep-rooted belief that eating the croissant would bring her peace and comfort.

In the end, your subconscious mind tends to win that battle. Remember, these are deep-rooted beliefs about who we are that have been wired in place over our entire lives! A few *yeah, buts* from your conscious mind ain't got nothin' on that!

All of this happened in a flash, most of it without Teri even realizing it. To her, it felt like she was utilizing free will: *do I want an apple or a croissant?*

What was *really* happening was an automatic response triggered by a subconscious belief: See croissant → Remember feeling of safe, loving home → Crave that feeling → Choose croissant.

That apple didn't stand a chance with Teri's conscious mind fighting her deep-rooted subconscious beliefs, without her even knowing.

Here's another example:

You look in the mirror.

That stimulus causes a flood of thoughts that aren't new. They're the same ones you've been telling yourself for the past twenty years:

My nose is too big.

Ew, that hair, though.

Why can't I have clear skin like Corrie from yoga? Fucking Corrie.

Where are they coming from? Maybe you grew up hearing about your genetically large nose. Maybe your sister was known for her long, shiny locks while you shamefully attempted to untangle comb after comb from your tangled mess. Maybe your mom and grandma always compared the clear skin your brother had to your acne-ridden pubescent face. Whatever was at the root, that simple glimpse in the mirror set off a chain reaction of negative thoughts and feelings, without you having to consciously do anything. You have a habit of thinking these negative thoughts after years of literally wiring your brain to respond this way!

Allow me to slip into my best infomercial voice here: "But wait! There's more!"

Here's the kicker: as is evident with our nose and hair thoughts above, oftentimes these pathways aren't even a conscious decision we've made! They come from things our parents told us or demonstrated growing up. They come from watching interactions go on around us. They come from the time in third grade mean Mr. Mitchell handed back your math tests in *descending order of grades* in front of the entire class, painfully remembering the embarrassment and shame you felt as you got your paper back dead last, along with his disapproving shake of his head, and every single pair of eyes in the classroom boring into your soul, filled with judgment. *Well, look at me now, Mr. Mitchell. Joke's on you!* Hypothetically, of course.

The point is, until we dig in and do the work of getting crystal clear on our current state of being, we're basically living the same day over and over again. We're the same person, with the same ingrained thoughts, and the same ingrained responses, leading to the same ingrained daily actions known as habits.

This is what it means when people say, "Change your thoughts, change your life." It's not some rainbows-and-unicorns-feel-good fluff.

It's neuroscience.

So, why the mini neuroscience lesson when this is supposed to be a book about health and fitness?

Because this is the foundation (that was totally a cement pun) of why you've never stuck with it in the past and how you *will* stick with it this time.

In chapter III, you got down on paper some of your limiting beliefs. Go back and reread them. Each one of those limiting beliefs triggers a response in you. Maybe you think, *I've started and stopped so many times. This is just going to be another disappointment*, and you give up on your new nutrition plan. Or maybe you believe *being overweight runs in my family*, and you stop your latest attempt at getting on a steady gym schedule.

Those responses are what's self-sabotaging your progress. They begin as thoughts you're telling yourself over and over again, move on to become deep-rooted beliefs, and, next thing you know, they've become who you are and what you do or do not do. They become your daily habits.

The beautiful part is this: Those neural pathways? We can control them. We can *choose* to create new ones that better serve us. We can *build habits that serve our goals* through conscious and consistent effort.

Pretty epic, right?

Let's talk about how.

ANYONE CAN LEARN ANYTHING.

Barring a major medical condition that's impaired your ability to process facts in the standard way, you can learn whatever the hell you want. Knitting, surfing, Portuguese, Kama Sutra, weightlifting, how to eat for your goals, whatever. Once you have the logistics, the *how* to do it and the *why it works*, it's simply a matter of practicing the movement/thought/activity over and over and letting your neural connections do their thang.

If your limiting beliefs from chapter III included anything logistic-related, pause right here and do a little happy dance. Then email a video to me because I can't watch other people get excited without dancing along with them. Seriously.

If you feel like you've tried every diet on the market and nothing has worked.

If you've spent ten of your thirty years on this earth in an endless internet search about fat loss and are still confused.

If you think the machines in the gym look like little green aliens who have come to Earth solely to laugh in your face and turn you into a what-not-to-do-in-the-gym meme, rest assured:

You can learn.

I'm pausing here for the dancing and the emailing.

This is a huge deal.

Not too long ago, science believed our brains were fixed. You were born a math person, or you weren't. You were born with musical talent, or you were one cane-around-the-neck away from being pulled off stage at all times. You were put on this earth to be a bodybuilder, or you were destined to follow in your family's footprints of obesity.

We now know what nonsense that is. *Hallelujah!*

Our brains are what's called *plastic. Brain plasticity* means that our brain has the ability to change. That by controlling, or not controlling, our thoughts and actions, we can literally rewire our brains.

In other words, not a math person? *Bullshit.* A good teacher, along with a lot of deep, concentrated practice, and you could be the next Einstein, with better hair, of course.

Not musically inclined? *Cue nope buzzer.* Some private lessons, a block of practice time each day, and a few years of consistency, you'll be booking your first gig at the Renaissance Festival, short pants and all. Fun fact: my first professional gig as a musician was at the South Florida Renaissance Festival. Fifty dollars for six hours of work: short pants, long herald trumpet, giant turkey drumstick and everything. It took me a half hour of practice, five days a week for two years to earn those short pants. Totally worth it.

Not a "fitness person"? *Try again.* Your brain is currently wired to believe this, being as how you've repeated that story over and over throughout your life. Add in some limiting beliefs from your family that you've heard since birth, and sprinkle on some hard "proof" each time you tried to lose fat and wound up gaining more, and you've got yourself a full-fledged, hardwired belief, my friend.

Now it's time to put what you learn in the pages ahead to use, do the work *consistently*, feed your mind some new, empowering beliefs, and rewire that brain for healthy, sustainable habits.

Your mom was right: you *are* beautiful, magical, and special. But you are not outside the laws of math and science. When you apply the tools in this book, they will work. For you, for me, for Karen in Accounting who's always doing the latest fad diet and trying to pull in anyone who will listen. Seriously, stop it, Karen.

Anyone can learn anything. That includes you when it comes to nutrition and fitness.

YOU CAN CHOOSE WHICH PATHWAYS YOU BUILD.

Repeat after me. Seriously. Say it out loud:

A belief is simply a thought I have repeated over and over until I've accepted it as truth.

Here's what that means. You may want to copy this one onto a

Post-It and stick it on your bathroom mirror for an early morning reminder:

Your truth is not the Truth.

I've always believed I was strong. Even when I was a kid, long before MindStrong existed, I thought I was tough, inside and out. I'd never lifted a weight, been on a treadmill, or done a push-up, but somehow, maybe it was my older brother constantly beating me up, maybe it was my dad's _Freimans never quit_ attitude, I believed I was a hard-ass kid.

This mindset served me as I got older.

It also fucked me up.

When it came to trying out for sports teams, starting a business, or lifting weights, I never doubted myself. I knew I was strong, so I knew I could handle whatever was put in front of me.

When it came to relationships, however, _whooooah_ boy. In my Tough Freiman story, strength came with the idea that vulnerability is weakness. That crying makes you weak. That expressing emotion is a sign of inferiority.

You can imagine how well that went over in relationships.

When the Universe decided it was time for me to learn one of my biggest lessons to date, it sent me Amanda. Into my life walked _the_ most in-tune-with-emotions human being I have ever met. This girl can read a person's energy in the time it takes me to get their name and inquire as to the number of dogs they have. Which, to my knowledge, is the appropriate way to greet potential new friends. In our house, we call it her superpower: she can *feel* what I'm feeling before I recognize it. Seriously, it's amazing. And slightly creepy.

I'd like to say I very quickly learned that being in touch with my emotions, being vulnerable, and having the confidence to open up and cry when it comes up, was a sign of strength. That wasn't the case. It took me years of practice and concentrated work to begin to accept these as my new truths. I continue to do the work to this day.

And it's no wonder the process is taking time! I had spent the first thirtysomething years of my life wiring my brain for the Freiman Way! This new, emotionally-in-tune, comfortable-with-vulnerability, feels-good-to-cry Rachel has been around for less time than half my wardrobe. She's got some work to do when it comes to rewiring that brain.

The point is this: *my* truth growing up, and for much of my adult life, was that vulnerability is a weakness. Because I didn't know any better, *and because the people around me as a child shared this belief so you* **know** *I was seeing and hearing affirmation of it on a daily basis,* that sucka became rooted deep. Like build-a-booty-squats deep.

But that doesn't mean that it's *Truth.*

It took meeting someone I love and respect, who lived and breathed this different truth, to show me that my truth was exactly that: *my* truth. It wasn't "just how life is." It was how I decided it was, and I told myself that thought over and over again, until it became a full-blown belief.

Whether it's *being vulnerable makes me weak, I'm not smart enough to go to college, I'm weak, I'm destined to be overweight* or *Who am I to be a stand-up comedian?* understand this:

The *only* reason you believe these things is because you've repeated them over and over until your brain has accepted them as truth. They are not Truth. They are *your* truth.

And we can rewrite our truth.

Go back to chapter III and pick your number one, go-to limiting belief. The one that, when you're honest with yourself, you revert to more often than the others.

Write it down. Now, really study it. Read it out loud. Repeat it over and over until the word *until* looks weird and you're questioning if it's really spelled like that and how has no one else noticed what a weird word that is before.

Think about three people in your life who inspire you, but don't share the same struggles you share. Let's be clear here: they have their own limiting bullshit and struggles; theirs just happen to be a different variety than yours. Would these three people accept your statement as Truth? If the answer is no, then you've just determined that this statement is *your* truth, not Truth.

For example:

> "I've tried every diet in the book and nothing has ever worked. Losing weight is impossible."

My friend Beth lost thirty pounds after struggling for years. She would not say that losing weight is impossible.

My uncle Steve is a hot mess when it comes to relationships, but man is he in shape! He would not say this is impossible.

Susan from my son's preschool is like Supermom. Somehow, she lost the baby weight in a few months, while running her own business. I bet she secretly drinks a lot 'cause no one has it all together like that, but, nonetheless, she wouldn't say that losing weight is impossible.

That's step one.

You've just shown yourself that this *isn't* Universal Law and it *is* changeable. It's simply a thought you've repeated to yourself over and over until it's become *your* truth, and we will change that. As we dive into actionable tools to literally rewire our brains for new, goal-serving thoughts, which lead to new, empowered beliefs, and, finally, new, productive daily habits, remember:

This isn't about standing in front of your bathroom mirror and screaming, "My body is a temple!" over and over until your neighbors spread the word and you soon find yourself living a life of celibacy.

It's about *consciously choosing* to create neural pathways that align with your goals and cementing them in place through focused, dedicated effort. It's about getting your mind aligned with your body to propel you forward rather than pull you back as it has been thus far.

It's doable, and it works—for you, for me, for Hot Mess Uncle Steve.

It's neuroscience.

CHARLIE VS. THE TRASH ROOM

So now that we know your beliefs are only *your* truth and not *the* Truth, how do we go about changing them? How do we move away from what we've trained ourselves to believe over years, or even decades? Simply *forcing* ourselves to change our thoughts won't work; we have to *replace* them with something.

Allow me to illustrate with Charlie versus the Trash Room.

When I first rescued my dog, Charlie, she was scared of *everything*. E.V.E.R.Y.T.H.I.N.G. Loud noises? *Check*. Things above her head? *Yup*. Shadows? *Uh huh*.

The day I took her out of the shelter, we went straight to a friend's house to get some puppy supplies. This friend lived in a beautiful high-rise apartment in Miami. Not bad for Charlie's first day of freedom, eh? The problem was, getting to this apartment meant parking in a huge parking garage, which, I quickly learned, was one of Charlie's biggest fears.

Now, if you're not a dog person, this next part won't have a fraction of the emotional impact I'm going for. If, however, you're a complete helicopter dog mom like me, grab some tissues.

After being gently coaxed out of the car, Charlie took one look around the enormous cement parking garage with her scared little puppy eyes open wide and laid her body as flat as it would go. I mean full-out "you'll never take me alive" mode: legs sprawled, eyes down, as-if-to-disappear-into-the-cement-flat, eliminating any option of walking her through this concrete hell. I had to carry her trembling forty-pound body through the garage, only to then be faced with the moving box from hell. Apparently, she was petrified of elevators as well. When we *finally* made it to the last barrier, a ridiculously heavy door that she was, of course, scared to go through, I made the Dog Mom Mistake of all Dog Mom Mistakes. Between trying to coerce her through the doorway, holding open that door that seriously weighed four times what a normal door should weigh, and nervously keeping an eye out for any passersby who might witness the event and think I'm torturing this poor, scared animal, I let go of the door too early. Charlie's little trembling paw got stuck in the door for a brief second, just long enough for her to let out a cry that haunts me to this day.

All in all, it was an emotionally scarring situation that neither of us would ever choose to repeat.

Fast forward three years. After living in our spacious South Florida home with its big yard, open driveway, and lack of scary parking garages, we made the decision to move to Northern California. Along with trading in endless humidity and early bird specials, we also found ourselves trading in the ease of the trash bin in our yard for a cement trash room that looked identical to, you guessed it, a smaller version of that evil parking garage from hell.

My helicopter mom ass wasn't putting my baby through that horror again.

So, the first time I had to stop in there with Charlie, I decided to make a game of it.

"Charlie!" I exclaimed in that voice saved solely for the privacy of when you're alone with your dog, "Wanna go on an *adventure*?!"

Charlie's tail is broken from her pre-shelter life, but, boy oh boy, did the little nub she can control wag frantically at those words! Tongue out, huge smile on her face, Charlie literally *bounded* around the corner and ran straight into the trash room. I tossed the poop bag with Charlie none the wiser to the anxiety she would have experienced in that room only three years earlier.

This has now become "our thing." Charlie *loves* the trash room. Whenever we turn the corner, her little eyes light up, waiting to hear the words, "Wanna go on an adventure?!" at which point she takes off with a mad dash to a room that, all things considered, *should* give her massive anxiety. I mean, Pavlov was pretty cool with his bell and his drooling, but did he get his dog excited about a trip to the trash room?!

While it's true that I'll look for any excuse to tell Charlie stories, there's a reason I'm sharing this. Something had happened in Charlie's past that caused her to be terrified of parking garages, and everything else, bless her soul. The way we undid this hard-wired fear was by *replacing* it with a new emotion: excitement. With *time and practice*, her response, a mad dash to paradise aka the trash room, became automatic and deeply ingrained, needing only the stimulus of rounding that corner.

As much as I believe my puppy to be the cutest, smartest, most perfect puppy on the face of the earth, I also have to believe that you are wildly more intelligent than she is. Which means your deep-rooted shit is engrained even deeper and your work to change those wirings is going to take more than me getting super excited and asking you if you "Wanna go on an adventure to the gym?!" But hot damn, would it be awesome if it were as easy as that.

The point is, your current thoughts about a situation trigger your current response. And all of these automatic, triggered responses have led to the state you are currently in, in every area of your life.

Let's say you associate the gym with feelings of judgment and insecurity. You feel anxious at the thought of it. But you know the gym is technically good for you. So, what do you do? You try to *force* change:

I hate the gym because I feel like everyone's staring at me and judging. It's uncomfortable. But my trainer says I have to go, so I probably should.

Does anything about that thought process scream success to you?! It's no wonder you canceled your membership within the first two months! As discussed in chapter II, our bodies and our minds are designed to avoid pain and seek pleasure. Forcing yourself to sit in your shit isn't the answer to getting comfortable.

Rewriting our thoughts around the situation is how we make change not only enjoyable but also sustainable:

I've always been afraid of the gym because I felt like everyone's staring at me and judging. I was uncomfortable. But you know what? I've realized that I'm there to make life changes. And I understand that every single person in there is there to accomplish his or her own goals. Plus, this time, I have a plan. I have instructions from my coach on which machines to use, and I'm gonna focus on that. I'm doing this for me, so let's go get my half hour in, knowing how great I'll feel for putting in the work.

Now we have a chance. A simple thought rewrite, and the chances of a new response skyrocket. Instead of focusing on the *fear* and on the *should*, you're focused on the *plan* and on your *why*.

If being that positive with yourself sounds foreign to you, or even a bit cheesy, or even a *lot* cheesy, go back to your work of Talking to Yourself like a Kindergartener. It works when you *continuously* do the work.

For now, understand this:

If you want to change your response (actions), you must begin by *consciously* changing your thoughts about the situation. By changing your thoughts about the situation, you can then build new responses that better serve your goals. Making the conscious choice of which pathways we build, and repeating this process over and over again, is how we build new, empowered habits.

And repeatedly building new, empowered habits is how we become the person we dream of being.

WE ARE WHAT WE REPEATEDLY DO

If our thoughts are causing these automatic responses, and we're having the same thoughts over and over, nearly every day of our lives, it's no wonder we feel stuck where we are.

We're doing the same shit over and over again, yet expecting ourselves to just snap out of it!

This is where *habit* becomes either your knight in shining armor or a face-eating zombie, your BFF or your archenemy.

Some habits are great for us.

I, for one, love that I've developed the habit of brushing my teeth every day. As do my peers.

One of the best habits I consciously built is being gentle with myself in my inner dialogue. It helps me push through challenging situations while being my best coach and teacher instead of my harshest critic. You now have the tools to create that habit too.

Some habits, typically those developed without that focused intent, aren't in our best interest. If we've spent years going from work to our car to our couch, that is now a daily habit.

We must *consciously work on* the habits we want to develop.

Remember, a belief is a thought we've repeated over and over until we've accepted it as truth. And that belief is leading you to respond in a certain way. And that response has been repeated over and over until your brain has put it on autopilot as your go-to whenever you have this thought. It's become a habit.

Let's take a common one:

> "I've started and stopped diets more times than I can count. It'll never stick!"

First, let's acknowledge that this is complete and utter bullshit. Not the starting and stopping part. I don't doubt you've done that. Most people have. (But never again. Remember, you wrote out a declaration in chapter III.) It's the second part of that statement that you've accepted as *Truth*, when it's really just *your* truth. You've been telling yourself this for years. It's a thought you've repeated over and over again until we can put it on its knee, tap it on both shoulders with a sword, and deem it A Belief.

So now the time comes to start Diet #5,473. As you read the instructions of what you can and can't eat for Diet #5,473, your belief alarm is going wild:

> "I've started and stopped diets more times than I can count. This will never stick!"

"I've started and stopped diets more times than I can count. This will never stick!"

"I've started and stopped diets more times than I can count. This will never stick!"

Tell me: how do you think Diet #5,473 is destined to work out for you?

But man oh man, we're not done yet!

Because when you quit Diet #5,473, which you inevitably will when you go in with the old approach and unconscious mindset, what happens? Well, now you have *more* proof!

"See?! I told you I've started and stopped diets more times than I can count and it'll never stick! Here's just one more example!"

And deeper and deeper the belief is rooted, and around and around the hamster wheel you go.

Repeated thoughts equal repeated responses equal repeated actions.

Repeated actions equal your current habits, which equal the state you are currently in.

So, how do we get off the wheel? How do we break the cycle? How do we rewire our brains with new, empowering beliefs and healthier habits that will result in the you that you dream of being? You've already done the first step. You've shone the light of awareness on *your current truths*, the limiting, bullshit beliefs that have been replaying in the back of your mind over and over all these years. Step two is to identify the actions and, eventually, habits, that these current limiting beliefs have led to.

Before we Put in the Work, I want to be clear about something: nowhere in my bio does it read "motivational speaker." I'm not here to simply say words that make you feel good while you're holding this book. I'm here to give you the tools you need to make lasting, sustainable change. This stuff works. But *only* when you put in the work. This book can either be yet another feel-good moment that's soon forgotten on the bookshelf and collecting dust, or it can be the one that makes it all click. Which one it becomes for you will be determined by how you approach it. Don't just read it. Do it.

Remember, I taught middle school for many, many years. Repeating myself until it sticks is deeply engrained:

Put. In. The. Work.

Put in the Work

Go back to chapter III and pick your poison. Take a limiting belief of your choosing from the list and write it down.

Now answer these questions. Don't filter. Don't edit. Verbally vomit all over the place.

- When I think this thought, I feel: Tight? Scared? Defeated? Frustrated?
- When I feel this way, what do I do? Bake cookies? Sit on the couch? Break shit? Cry?
- Has this thought and the action it produces led to a habit that gets me closer to or further from my goals? Why?
- Am I ready to change this belief? You don't need to know how yet. You don't even need to believe you can yet. If I could wave a magic dumbbell and change it for you, are you ready? (Answering Yes or No will do.)

Now go back and do this for each limiting belief you wrote down in chapter III, as well as any new ones that are coming up for you.

CHAPTER VI

REDEFINE FEAR

"People have a hard time letting go of their suffering. Out of a fear of the unknown, they prefer suffering that is familiar."

—THICH NHAT HANH

YOU, ME, AND CALVIN

I'm about to tell you something that's going to cause one of two reactions:

1. You might get insulted. "What did you just say to me?! How dare you!" type of pissed.
2. You might shrug it off, based on religious beliefs or basic self-confidence, and insist that this does not apply to you.

It does.

What I'm about to tell you applies to everyone, from you, to me, to the Dalai Lama himself. In fact, the only reason you might not think of the Dalai Lama as being in the same category as you or me when it comes to this is because the dude wakes up at 3:00 a.m. and meditates for hours to train his mind, *in large part because this fact applies to him.* Don't worry. Nowhere in this chapter will you be asked to spend six hours on a meditation mat. Our work will be powerful, though much less time-consuming.

Nonetheless, if your classification in this world is that of a human, this fact remains:

You have a caveman brain.

I'll pause while the indignation passes and the insults fly.

Allow me to clarify what this *isn't*:

This *isn't* me telling you that your intelligence is limited to banging on your chest, barely walking upright, and tearing meat off large bones with your teeth. It also isn't to be confused with the popular "Caveman Diet," a fad diet whereupon the idea is to eat like our caveman ancestors in an attempt to live longer and be healthier. Um, how long did the average caveman live? Thankfully that fad diet is now becoming more or less, wait for it, extinct.

Whatever your beliefs about how we came to be, the fact remains that we have caveman brains. This isn't about evolution from a theoretical or religious standpoint. It's about science.

Over time, as in thousands and millions of years' time, species adapt. Whether it's lizards growing stickier feet to be better able to climb trees, owls changing color to blend into their surroundings for survival, or bedbugs growing thicker shells to better resist pesticides (yes, this is a thing), science has shown that many living creatures currently inhabiting our earth do not take the same form as the ones that were walking, crawling, or flying around when they originally crashed this party. They've adapted. Survival of the fittest and all.

Humans have done a bang-up job of this as well. We now walk totally upright on two legs. *Woohoo!* We can communicate in more ways than grunting, despite what many people at the gym would lead you to believe. All around, we're adapting to better fit the world in which we live.

However, a quick look at our brain during times of stress shows the following activity:

A threat is perceived. A part of your brain called the amygdala sounds the alarm to your hypothalamus, letting it know shit's gettin' real and it's about to go down. The hypothalamus rallies the squad, or, in this case, the sympathetic nervous system, kickin' that sucka into high gear and getting your adrenaline going. With adrenaline comes faster breathing, increased heart rate and blood pressure, and even the constriction of key blood vessels to get blood into larger muscle groups so you can flex on 'em. In other words, everything you'd need for a good ol' fashioned throw down should you choose to fight rather than flee. This reaction to stress is biological. We all have it. And it's the same one experienced by our long-lost ancestor, Calvin the Caveman. When it comes to stress, we haven't yet evolved. We have caveman brains.

Here's the good news: that brain is also the reason you're reading this book. I don't just mean because it's processing the information you need to read these words; I mean because it's extremely difficult to read if you're dead.

And that's what your and Calvin the Caveman's brain was designed to do: *keep you alive.*

Let's be super clear on this point:

The *single role* of your caveman brain is to keep you alive.

Not happy.

Not flourishing.

Not kickin' ass and takin' names.

Alive.

Calvin the Caveman lived in a very different world than you and I. Instead of hitting snooze five times on his smartphone before squinting one eye open to quickly scan emails and ensure his boss hasn't started bombarding his inbox at the ungodly hour of 5:00 a.m., his morning routine included getting his caveman booty off that cave floor at the first crack of light to start hunting and foraging before he and his family became saber-tooth tiger breakfast.

A glimpse into ol' Cal's day might look something like this:

Sun peeks up behind a hill

Twig snaps nearby

Saber-tooth tiger peeks its head around a rock

Calvin, bolting upright and grabbing a hand-carved spear: "Tiger!"

Cathy the Cavewoman, Calvin's wife: "I'm sure it's nothing, dear, come back to bed."

Calvin: "Nothing?! There's a freakin' saber-tooth tiger mere feet from us, ready to pounce on our kids and make them its breakfast! Seriously?! Nothing?! This could be the end of our family! How can you be so relaxed?! Cover me. I'm going in!"

Cathy: "Oh, Calvin, you're always jumping to the worst-case scenario. But OK, dear, whatever you want. Just be careful." *Falls back to sleep*

Imagine what's going on in Calvin's body at this point: his heart rate and blood pressure are increased, he's breathing faster, his blood vessels in certain parts of his body are constricted, forcing more blood to go to larger muscle groups. He's in full-out fight-or-flight mode. His body is responding in a way that's preparing him to either run to safety or prepare to fight. Because this is a biological response, one built for fight-or-flight, the symptoms are more or less universal.

Now, let's imagine modern day Cal, rolling over on his comfy, adjustable mattress and hitting snooze on his smart phone for the third time. Oh, how times have changed.

After thirty minutes of "just-five-more-minutes" snoozing, Calvin cracks open one sleep-crusted eye and scans his email. With a sinking feeling in his gut, he sees what he was dreading: an email marked urgent from his boss.

Email: "Calvin:"

Calvin's Mind: *Calvin?! Not even a "Hi Calvin?" Not a "Dear Calvin?!" Ugh, this can't be good.*

Email: "It has come to my attention that there's a concern over the safety of one of our construction cranes."

Calvin's Mind: *Come to your attention?! I've been telling you that for months! This guy never listens to me! What am I, dinosaur food?!*

Email: "I'd like to set up a meeting to discuss this situation for tomorrow morning at 8:00 a.m. in my office. See you there."

Calvin's Mind: *8:00 a.m.?! That's in twenty minutes! I'll never make it in time! I'll be fired! I've been telling him about this issue for at least three months, and suddenly it's so urgent that I need to check my email every evening just to know about an 8:00 a.m. meeting?? And now I could lose my job if I don't get there in time! And if I lose my job, what will my family do?! We'll starve! We'll be out on the streets! This is a disaster!*

What's going on with Calvin's body right about now? It's a safe guess that his heart rate and blood pressure are increased, his breathing is faster, and the blood vessels in certain parts of his body are constricted, forcing more blood to go to larger muscle groups.

Sound familiar?

While being eaten by a wild animal and emails from a micro-managing boss are both stressful, I think it's fair to label them as different types of stress. One is psychological. An email can be stressful, annoying, or even upsetting, but the act of reading it will not cause you physical harm. In the extremely rare case that a physical reaction does occur, in the form of a panic attack or even heart attack, it wasn't the email itself that brought on the physical condition. It was your *thoughts* about the email. In other words, that email did not reach into your body, pinch those coronary arteries closed, restrict blood flow to your heart, and physically induce a heart attack. Instead, you read the email, had a thought or fifty about its contents, and interpreted those thoughts according to what you believe they mean. All of this caused a physical reaction within your body that, when mixed with your current level of health, brought on the heart attack.

The email was the catalyst, not the physical cause.

A saber-tooth tiger ten feet away, however, is a pretty damn clear cause.

If our ol' pal Calvin were to be torn to bits by Sammy the Saber-tooth, well, there's little arguing about the cause. It wasn't his feelings about Sammy or his interpretation of the interaction that lead to his death. It was pretty clearly Sammy's saber-tooth teeth ripping him to pieces that caused Calvin's tragic demise.

When it comes to our caveman brain, it doesn't know, nor does it care, if the stress is psychological or physical.

Before you go getting pissed at your poor caveman brain for being more dramatic than a reality TV star, keep in mind that it's just doing its evolutionary job of keeping you alive. And that's a great thing! I personally love being alive. I hope to do more of it. The issue is, we no longer live in Calvin the Caveman's world of saber-tooth tigers.

Let's be clear: we do all have moments of *danger*, immediate physical threat. I once looked the wrong way for the subway train and missed being decapitated by all of ten seconds. Thankfully, my caveman brain was scanning the situation and heard what was happening in time for me to pull my head back, and here we are today. I've also narrowly dodged being hit by a car on multiple occasions. While writing this has made me contemplate just how many times this has happened, and perhaps I should stop walking around with headphones on, the point remains: I am thankful for my caveman mind. It is because of its constant scanning that I'm here writing this rather than headless or caught in endless hit-and-run lawsuits.

Yet, *constant* physical threat is not the reality for most of us. The majority of our day is not spent hunting and gathering or scanning for wild beasts lurking behind bushes. We may scan for an annoying coworker near the water cooler, but he won't kill us, though it certainly feels like death by annoyance could be a thing. The majority of our danger in a day comes from psychological threat, not physical threat.

This often leads to the question of why it's "so difficult" to be positive. It often seems as if our default mental state is worry, stress, and negativity. The answer is part biological and a whole lot of habit. In psychology, it's known as the negativity bias.[8] Left unchecked, or more specifically, *untrained*, our nature is to process and cling to the negative rather than the positive. Because of that caveman brain, we are wired to be on the lookout for bad shit.

What we need to understand is that we're not *destined* to be negative. You've just spent the last twenty, thirty, forty, fifty, or sixty years letting your caveman brain call the shots. It's been scanning, stressing, and signaling threats to your body at the slightest chance of harm, whether it be a text message or a semi-truck. And as we know from our work with habits, neurons that fire together, wire together.

This means that your caveman brain has had the same worried thoughts *so* many times that it is now literally *wired to worry*.

Through *conscious effort* we can rewire our brain to look for the positive in life, rather than constantly scanning for lurking tigers or other signs of threat. We can teach ourselves to discern between danger, immediate physical harm, and psychological threat or inconvenience, use its alarm as a sign, *redefine* it, and go on with our bad selves.

YOUR INTERNAL SEARCH HISTORY

Our body is a master at communicating with us.

Like a toddler pulling on his mother's shirt and crying, "Mom! Mom! Mom!" until she pays attention, it's constantly giving us signs as to what's going on internally. But, like that busy mom, we're often too caught up in daily life to pay attention.

When your caveman brain senses danger, any kind of danger, it sends you a message to let you know it's time to sharpen up.

That message is sent in the form of *fear.*[9]

Fear is the underlying roadblock of all those unfilled dreams you're suppressing. Why? We've misinterpreted what fear means. Well, misinterpreted is a generous word. Fear, driven by that caveman brain and its heroic effort to keep you alive, has thrown every trick in the book to get you out of what it has deemed to be harm's way. And we've fallen for it. Every. Single. Time.

How it does this is actually quite impressive, in a sneaky-little-bastard kind of way. Fear knows you better than anyone in the universe. Better than your spouse, your mother, even your bestie. It even knows those thoughts hidden deep in your subconscious, the ones you feel but haven't fully acknowledged because they're too big and scary. The thoughts of *What if my business fails and I can't support my family and they leave me and I die alone?* Or, *What if I put myself out there and ask her on a date and she laughs in my face, deeming me undatable to everyone else at work and I wind up a social outcast, destined to die in my apartment, surrounded only by my cats?* Even if you've never fully followed the unraveling thread to its root, Fear knows.

And that's exactly what it will use in the name of keeping you alive.

Imagine seeing your daughter playing in the middle of the street. In the distance, you can see an oncoming speeding car. The driver is texting and has no clue that your entire world is a little farther up the road and you're too far away to run to her in time.

You call out to her, "Amelia, get out of the road, baby!"

She looks at you, shakes her head, and continues playing.

So you try again, more urgently: "Amelia! GET OUT OF THE STREET **NOW**!"

Amelia looks at you, looks at her toys, hesitates as she weighs her options, then turns her back to you and continues playing.

At this point, you're frantic. The only thing you care about in the entire world is getting your baby to safety.

What do you do? Anything.

"Amelia, if you come here right now, I'll give you candy and ice cream and we'll go to the movies and I'll buy you three puppies!"

Well, now you've got Amelia's attention and she's on the move.

Did it matter that you had to pull every trick in the book to get her there? Not in the moment. Your priority was to keep her alive, and you did that successfully. Mission accomplished.

The same rule applies to Fear, minus the puppies and ice cream. When it comes to keeping you alive, it will throw every trick in the book to keep you right where it thinks you should be: in your comfort zone, where you're safe. The issue is, Fear is not using logic to determine if the threat is an oncoming car or a nagging boss.

Its only measure of threat is experience. In its world, anything new equals threat, and threat equals death.

Fear works a lot like your computer. I, for one, would be lost without my computer's search history. From remembering specific websites to finding products I was debating whether or not to buy for two full weeks, clicking that little icon and being able to look back at what I had previously viewed is invaluable. Not to mention that my computer can even *anticipate* what I'm about to search for based on my previous activity. This collection of past experiences is how our computer keeps track of our journey into the cyber world. Fear does the same thing in its attempt to keep you alive.

You set off on a new venture, and the first thing Fear does is scroll through its search history, its database of past experiences:

Have you ever, in fact, started Linda's Canine Cardigans, an online business dedicated to adorable fancy sweaters for dogs?

Scrolls through search history

You haven't?

Death.

Oh, you're taking Suzy Squatsalot from the gym out on a first date?

Have you ever, in fact, been on a date with a girl whose booty is literally implied in her last name?

Scrolls through search history

Never?

Death.

A gym routine, you say? We're not going to go straight from work to the couch to find out who's staying and who's going this week on our favorite reality dating show? Instead, we're going to go to a weird-smelling place with lots of dangerous machines and pushing ourselves to do physical work after a long day? Have we done this before?

Scrolls through search history

Oh! We have! And we quit after two weeks. OK, I'll let you have this one for a few weeks, then be sure to remind you that our place is in the comfort zone of our couch. Because too much of this activity and I wouldn't recognize our life anymore. *Death.*

If you've started and stopped countless diets before, you're all too familiar with this Fear jujitsu and its attempts to pin you down and hold you where you are using every move in the book. Fear is sneaky. It knows that, just like your failed attempts to get little Amelia out of harm's way, a simple "Please don't do this" ain't gonna cut it when it comes to your stubborn ass. It knows you well enough to know that when you're set on something, you will do it, come hell or high water.

So, it pulls out all the stops: the past failures, the insecurities, the family, everything and anything that could potentially get you back to your comfort zone. Just like bribing little Amelia with ice cream and puppies, it does what it has to do to get you to safety and avoid what it interprets as death.

I had a client, Taylor, whose caveman brain loved to use her two-year-old as her fear pressure point.

This was a conversation Taylor and I had when we first started working together:

Taylor: "I want to lose the thirty pounds I gained after Jackson was born, but it's just not possible."

Me: "Why isn't it possible?"

Taylor: "First of all, I've tried for over a year now. I lose ten pounds, then gain back fifteen."

Me: "Sounds like we need a new approach. Why else isn't it possible?"

Taylor: "I just don't have time. Jackson's home with my husband all day. I get home from a full day of teaching just in time to put him to bed, but then I'm exhausted. The thought of going to the gym after a full day like that just isn't realistic. Plus, I haven't seen my husband all day, so even if I could make it to the gym at that point, it'd be selfish of me to go."

Me: "Is that a conversation you've had with your husband or something you've decided on your own?"

Taylor: "We haven't actually talked about any of this. He'd probably just tell me to do whatever I had to do, knowing I wouldn't stick with it. I never have before. Why would this time be any different? It won't and everyone knows it. My parents and his parents are all overweight. It's in our genes. I don't know why I even put so much effort into thinking about this. I'll never change. This is who I am."

Let's take a glimpse into Taylor's search history:

Has she tried fitting a gym routine into her day? Nope. That's new. And scary. *Death.*

Has she ever balanced time with her child and time with her husband with time for herself to feel happy and healthy? No ma'am. That's uncharted territory. *Death.*

Has she tried losing weight in the past? Yup. But don't worry, it never lasts. So, we'll let her try, temporarily. Then right back to the comfort zone we go.

Has *anyone* in her family made a change in lifestyle and gotten their health in check? Absolutely not. Well then, this is totally new for everyone. *Certain death.*

As we can see, Fear isn't tapping Taylor on the shoulder, saying, *Um, excuse me. I'm concerned that if you start a new, empowered lifestyle, it's going to be an adjustment for your whole family, so perhaps we should stay put in our comfort zone.*

Hell no. That sucker's pullin' out all the stops to get her to stay put:

> *Get healthy?! You?! How many times are we gonna do this dance? You know you'll just quit in a couple of weeks. But, lemme get this straight: you have a baby at home, a husband taking care of him all day while you work with other people's kids, and now you want to come home, see them both for an hour, then go take time for yourself so you can look a certain way?! How selfish and egotistical can you get?! And it's all in vain! Your entire family is overweight. This is your destiny! Embrace it and just be a good wife and mom. Be practical. Stay home and live the life you're destined for.*

Every single feeling of guilt, feeling of failure, and feeling of defeat that Taylor's experiencing is Fear, driven by her caveman brain, attempting to keep her where it knows she'll be safe. Same life. Same routine. Same Taylor. When you start to get brutally honest with yourself, you will begin to see where your caveman brain and, by extension, Fear, has convinced you to stay in your comfort zone.

I say brutally honest because, remember: Fear is sneaky.

Besides pushing on your deepest, darkest pressure points, it's also convincing you that going back to your comfort zone is for your own good. The rationale for why it's not feasible to start your business, the excuse that family genes are the reason you're overweight, the perceived "selfishness" of making yourself a priority, it all makes sense, doesn't it? It seems logical. Maybe Fear is right after all and staying put is the wisest thing to do.

It's not.

The issue is, up until now, we've taken Fear's word as Gospel. We believed it to be Truth and followed accordingly. As we're about to learn, when we identify the feeling of fear, acknowledge it, thank it for attempting to do its only job of keeping us safe, and *use it in a new, productive way,* then, and only then, can we move forward into the life we dream of.

REDEFINE FEAR

Saying you don't feel fear is bullshit.

Anyone who claims to never experience the feeling of fear is claiming to defy the biological structure of human beings. When checking into hotels, Amanda researches exit routes and evacuation plans like a boss. I assume everything is fine always, until I see a butterfly trying to land on me, in which case I freak out and bolt for one of her perfectly planned escape routes.

Different people, different threats, different fear. But, at some point, we all experience fear. It's biological.

We are not here to "bust through fear." Despite the image of your stereotypical gym trainer, I am not a believer in getting in people's faces, screaming, "NO FEAR!!" as they do burpees until their legs collapse beneath them.

I am a believer in acknowledging Fear and redefining what it means.

If Fear is the distress signal from our caveman brain that what we're about to do does not exist in our brain's search history, then Fear is a sign that we're onto something new, big, and exciting. In other words:

Fear is a sign that you're onto something badass.

In the past, we've allowed Fear to run the show. We took its presence to mean that what we're about to do isn't big and badass, but big and scary. We let it push on our deep, dark pressure points until we yelled mercy and retreated back into our comfort zone.

Not anymore.

With our new definition of Fear comes new power. Once we recognize Fear for what it is, a sign that we're embarking on something new, and recognize *why* it's showing up, our caveman brain's way of keeping us alive by convincing us to retreat into our comfort zone, we can then change our relationship with fear.

Let's go back to Taylor and her guilt-ridden, fear-based thoughts.

Fear: *Get healthy?! You?! How many times are we gonna do this dance? You know you'll just quit in a couple of weeks.*

New, empowered Taylor: *Oh hey, Fear! I see you're worried about a lifestyle shift. Thank you. Seriously. I know your intention is to keep me safe, and I appreciate you. Yes, I did try in the past and I gave up. I recognize that I was attempting to do this based on restriction, which I now know isn't sustainable. This time, I have a coach, I'm getting educated, and I'm set up for success.*

Fear: *Lemme get this straight: you have a baby at home, a husband taking care of him all day while you work with other people's kids, and now you want to come home, see them both for an hour, then go take time for yourself so you can look a certain way?! How selfish and egotistical can you get?!*

New, empowered Taylor: *I realize you're worried that taking time for myself will lead to a new Taylor you don't recognize, and I know how scary change can be. But I also know that showing up as my healthiest, most energetic self is the single best thing I can do for my family. My husband is a supportive man and a wonderful father. It's why I married him and had a child with him! I know that an open and honest talk will get him onboard to figure out a plan that works for all of us. I know you're scared of this change, Fear. I recognize you want to keep me safe. But this is for the best.*

Fear: *And it's all in vain! Your entire family is overweight. This is your destiny! Embrace it and be a good wife and mom. Be practical. Stay home and live the life you're destined for.*

New, empowered Taylor: *No, this is my comfort zone because it is what I've been around my whole life. Which means it's time for a change and time to set an example for my family that change is possible. The life I'm destined for includes the healthiest version of myself. Thank you for the warning that this is new and scary, but I've got it from here.*

Taylor went from finding reasons why she couldn't make a change and letting fear talk her back into her comfort zone, to redefining what fear meant to her, a warning that this was new and scary, and using it to make sure a plan was in place for this uncharted territory so she could *keep going.*

By doing so, Taylor stuck with her new routine, and her husband supported her along the way. In fact, taking control of her health inspired him to do the same, resulting in an arrangement where her mom watched Jackson while they spent quality time together at the gym. Their shared goal only made their relationship stronger and allowed for greater accountability and more support at home.

This is what it means to redefine fear.

Fear no longer controls you. It no longer stops you from livin' large. It's now simply a sign, a flashing light, signaling that you're in new, uncharted territory. It's telling you that it's time to come up with a plan and continue on.

Fear is not a bad thing. On the contrary, it can help us to keep a good balance of "head in the clouds" versus "feet on the ground." It reminds us that this *is* new, and new can be scary. We need a plan. We might need to do some research, or a lot of it. We may need to ask questions. And then more questions. And then even more questions. We may need to go back to school. To get a second job. To quit a job. To have a discussion we've been avoiding.

Because Fear knows us so well, it's using pressure points that it knows are in that subconscious mind of yours. It's not randomly making shit up to scare you; it's using your deep, dark worries and bringing them to the surface for you. That's invaluable! You now know what to focus on when it comes to making a plan. It's showing you where to start with actionable steps so you can move forward.

Like Taylor, maybe you *have* quit more diets than you can count. That doesn't mean you shouldn't try again. But it *does* mean that trying a different method would be in your best interest. *Thanks, Fear.*

You might feel guilty asking your spouse for "you time" when they've been home with the kids all day. That doesn't mean you shouldn't have the conversation. It means it's time to dig deep into what limiting belief has led you to feel that taking care of you has been placed on the back burner. *Thank you, Fear.*

Your whole family might be overweight. That doesn't mean you're destined to be as well. It means it's time to break the cycle and set the example, using a solid plan and prioritizing taking care of yourself. *You really are the best, Fear. Thank you.*

When we take control of Fear, it no longer controls us. When we redefine what it means, we learn to use it as a tool.

It becomes a warning sign.

A fever tells us something's out of balance within our body. We don't give up on life and call it quits. We eat our vegetables, drink some tea, and go to the doctor if necessary. Thirst tells us we're dehydrated. We don't throw in the towel and prepare to wither away. We drink some water. Fear tells us we're about to do something big and new. We don't stop. We hear the message, learn what needs to be learned, and proceed.

This is powerful stuff.

Redefining fear is one of the most important tools you can use when it comes to creating a new, healthy lifestyle because any lifestyle change is an opportunity for Fear to run rampant. Health is not only a major change, which we know equates to death in our caveman brain, but it's also a major change that most of us have struggled with, unsuccessfully, most of our lives. In other words, our caveman brain has a plethora of search history content from which to choose.

The key is to take control.

First, acknowledge Fear. Thank it for having your best interest of staying alive at heart. Then let it know that you've got it from here. Message received, but now you're taking the reins.

Redefining Fear takes brutal honesty with yourself. We need to first shine the light of awareness on what's actually happening in each area of our life, acknowledge where Fear has a hold on us, redefine what it's telling us, and then step forth onto our new path with confidence and freedom.

When my client Jen came to me, she had tried nearly every diet out there (including the Caveman Diet!) and felt defeated. I introduced her to one of my favorite exercises, Redefining Fear, which you too will have the opportunity to do in the Put in the Work section. Through this exercise, we learned what was really going on: Fear was telling her she's not cut out for this. Fear was keeping her in her comfort zone.

We started by listing an area of health where Jen felt stuck in column one. Once we got it down, the second column was for the current reason she was telling herself as to *why* she was stuck. *This* is where the digging deep happens. When you read over column two, everything makes sense. It seems logical. Jen could easily go through life and rationalize why column one was the way it was, using the rationale of column two. But Jen now knew better. In column three, she identified what role Fear was playing in this rationale. She got 100 percent clear on how Fear has been holding her back so that, in column four, she could redefine that relationship with a clear plan of how to move forward.

COLUMN I: WHERE I FEEL STUCK	COLUMN II: WHY I FEEL STUCK	COLUMN III: ROLE OF FEAR	COLUMN IV: REDEFINE FEAR
Weight Loss	I feel like I'm destined to be overweight for the rest of my life. I make progress and then I regress big-time. It's like two steps forward, five steps back. I don't know if it's my genetics or my metabolism, but I feel like this just isn't for me, like I'm just destined to be permanently overweight. My whole family is overweight, so I should probably just accept it as who I am.	I recognize that Fear is holding me back from sticking with my weight loss goals. Every single time I "mess up," that little voice kicks in, telling me I'm kidding myself thinking it'll be any different this time. I'm afraid of failing yet again. I'm afraid to start, only to be disappointed yet again. I'm afraid of having another conversation with my family about my goals, only to fall short yet again. I always thought I was incapable of this, but, when I get honest with myself, it's me that's holding me back. My caveman mind is throwing every trick in the book at me to keep me in my comfort zone, to keep me as the me I've always known. I'm giving up because I'm afraid to fail.	Now that I see Fear, I can't unsee it. Every time that little voice tells me I'm kidding myself for thinking I can change, I automatically think, "Oh, hey there, Fear!" So, it's time to redefine what Fear means to me. This lifestyle change is new and scary. I have tried countless times and been disappointed. I have had countless conversations with my family and fallen short on the goals that I shared with them. But I now have three things I never had before: an education on how this works, a coach for accountability and support, and my eyes wide open to the role Fear is playing in all this. From now on, I'm redefining what Fear means on this journey. It no longer gets to dictate what I can or can't do. It's simply a sign that I'm onto something new and big. It's a sign that I'm stepping out of my comfort zone, which is exactly what I need to do to be successful on this journey. I will thank it for giving me a heads-up that the steps I'm taking are new and huge, and then tell Fear that it's done its part and can go now. I've got it from here.

This works for everything and, when you dig deep, can unleash the potential in all areas of your life. Any time you embark on a major lifestyle change, from starting a business to losing weight, Fear is going to be there with you, attempting to take over the driver's seat. By putting in the work, you can redefine the message it's sending you and take back control.

Put in the Work

Grab your journal and draw four columns. Make sure to give yourself plenty of room so you can completely verbally vomit all over the page. It's important to get it all out.

I encourage you to go back and repeat this exercise with any and every area of your life where you're currently feeling less than 1,000 percent fulfilled; just be sure to focus on only one area at a time.

Label the first column **Where I Feel Stuck**

Label the second column **Why I Feel Stuck**

Label the third column **Role of Fear**

Label the fourth column **Redefine Fear**

In the first column, list the area where you're feeling stuck. This will be a short statement, not a full paragraph. It might be weight loss, muscle growth, nutrition, or any other area you're not feeling your best.

The second column is where you get brutally honest. Let it all out. Why do you feel stuck? What stories have you been telling yourself? Don't judge; just get honest and write it all down. What's keeping you here?

The third column is where we dig deep. Knowing what you now know about Fear, what's *really* going on? What role is Fear playing? Why are you *really* stuck when you release the stories you've been holding onto and recognize the role of Fear? Write it all down.

The fourth column is our step into our new life. It's time to redefine fear. You can speak directly to Fear, or you can write out a plan. Either way, how will you go forth knowing what you now know has *really* been holding you back? What role will you allow Fear to play in your life and how will you take control over it? You're the boss now. Let Fear know.

CHAPTER VII

LIFE IS ENERGY

The universal order and the personal order are nothing but different expressions and manifestations of a common underlying principle.
—MARCUS AURELIUS

My friend Victoria is forty-five and has three kickass daughters, a loving husband of twenty-one years, a dog, two lizards, a frog, and no time for herself. She's also almost single-handedly responsible for why I started MindStrong Fitness.

Victoria and I taught together back when I was a middle school music teacher. Over the years, she had slowly gained weight. When she and I met, she had hit that oh-so-familiar point of *how did this happen?!*

"Rachel," she told me one day in school, "I don't understand what happened. I used to be the young, fit one! Now I look in the mirror and barely recognize myself. Like, I'm a *mom*. And not just a mom, a mom with a *mom bod*! I can't believe what I see, and I definitely can't believe I let myself get like this. I keep telling myself I need to do something about it, but then I'm too tired, or the kids have to go somewhere, or my husband's away for work, so I'm on mom duty. I just feel...stuck."

After a few more conversations like this, I asked Victoria if she'd like to try going to the gym with me. She responded that she'd like to but was nervous about it. She didn't know where to start. When she did occasionally exercise, it was dance-based cardio, which she loved, but not enough to do consistently. I often went to the gym in the morning before work, so I told her to pick a day and meet me there, and I would handle the rest.

Well, apparently, three teenaged daughters led to some pent-up energy that needed to come out somewhere and, man-oh-man, did Victoria take it out on those weights! She was a *beast* in the gym! Any exercise I gave her to do, she *crushed*. Grunting, pushing herself to lift heavier, full-out powerhouse mode activated.

But this isn't some tale of Victoria finding her true calling in bodybuilding. Having never lifted weights before, she got tired quickly, frustrated that she couldn't lift more, and had three breakdowns in the first hour about how disappointed she was in letting her weight get to this point.

And she had a fantastic workout.

Late that night, I got the following text:

> "I can barely move my arms. Everything hurts. I feel amazing. Can I come with you tomorrow?"

While Victoria didn't show up every single morning, she was there enough to begin to form a habit and start seeing results. Every night, she would text me about what body part was now sore and how great it was to feel herself getting stronger. It was an amazing feeling to hear her talk about her results.

One day, Victoria was talking about her new workout routine. This time, however, the conversation wasn't focused on how great her newfound muscle soreness was but on her life outside of the gym.

> "You know what's crazy? Since I started working out, I feel like a better partner to my husband. I'm just...I don't know...happier. I have more energy when I get home. I feel good about myself so I don't freeze up when he tries to put his hand around my waist, worrying about the 'spare tire' he might feel. I see it with my kids too. I'm more patient simply 'cause I'm not dragging when I get home as I had been for years. Hell, I even see it in my classroom! My students feel it! You know I had a kid ask me if everything's OK the other day. When I asked him why, he responded, 'I don't know...you just seem...happy lately.' Can you imagine?! Three weeks ago, I avoided every mirror I walked by. Truth be told, I've avoided mirrors for the past ten years. Ugh. Saying that out loud, I hear how sad that is. But it's true. Now I catch myself catching a glimpse to see if I can see some definition in my arms! It's just unreal how amazing I feel in my everyday life just by putting in this hour each day."

Well, that was it for me. When people describe love at first sight, that moment when you just *know* something was meant to be, this was mine. What Victoria had described was exactly what I wanted to help every single human being achieve. Because I know that every single human being *can* achieve it. Even if they don't believe it yet.

Victoria's experience sums up what I consider to be the most important part of getting your health in check. Big muscles are fun. Knowing you can carry all twelve bags of groceries in one trip feels amazing. Your health is incredibly important. But the underlying reason why getting your fitness and nutrition in check changes how you show up in the world is because it drastically changes your energy.

And life is all about energy.

QUANTUM PHYSICS AND YOUR BADASS LIFE

When most people hear the words *energy* and *vibes* (vibrations), it's followed by a groan, an exaggerated eye roll, and thoughts of hippies, sandals, peace signs, and rainbows. What energy and vibes *really* come down to, however, is the branch of science dedicated to nature in its smallest form: quantum physics.

Within quantum physics, scientists have discovered that when you break an atom down until it can't be broken down any further, 99.9 percent of every atom is not physical matter—it's energy.[10] If you just glossed over that sentence, go back and reread that. *It's a really big freakin' deal.*

As we learned in grade school science, everything in life is made up of atoms. What we now know is that atoms are not made up primarily of physical matter, but energy. Think about what that means! You, me, the car you drive, the trees outside, that dream house you can't stop fantasizing about, the Chihuahua next door that sounds like it swallowed a squeak toy every time it barks, we are all made up of *energy*.

If we left the conversation there, I would hope that's enough to understand why having shit tons of energy is important. We *exert* energy. We *need* energy. We *are* energy.

But we haven't even tapped into the most important part of this: the concept that *like attracts like.*

In music, we have something called a tuning fork. A tuning fork is a small piece of metal that, when tapped, is designed to give off a particular tone. This tone is created through the vibration of the metal causing sound waves. A typical tuning fork is A440Hz, which produces the note A.

Buckle in. This shit's about to get real.

Let's say you took that A440 tuning fork into a room filled with tuning forks. It's like a band director's hell in there, but, nonetheless, there you are. Some of the tuning forks in the room are A440 Hz. Some are set to other notes: 288 Hz (the note D), 320 Hz (the note E), etc. You tap your A440 tuning fork. What do you think happens? The tuning forks set to other frequencies do nothing. They're just hanging out, minding their tuning fork business. The other A440 tuning forks in the room, however, start sounding! The simple act of setting off your A440 tuning fork set them off as well! Why? Because a rule of quantum physics exists that *like attracts like.*

We've seen it said a million ways in a million memes:

Your vibe attracts your tribe.

Good vibes only.

Think positive, be positive.

While it's easy to scroll past Ashley the Social Media Influencer's eleventh social media post about positivity, it's hard to brush past the fact that quantum physics has confirmed that this is science:

Since atoms, at their smallest form, are energy, and since we are all made up of atoms, we are, in our simplest form, energy. Because like attracts like, we *literally* attract back the energy we put out.

That, my friends, is science in its most mind-blowing form.

GOOD VIBES ONLY

Think of it this way: if we could physically *see* vibration with our bare eyes, we would see that everything around us emits energy.

You don't need the title Dr. before your name to understand the basics of how this would work. Becki in HR that either eats pancakes topped with edible glitter each morning or has cracked the code to brewing her own Happy Bubbly Giddy Potion? *High vibe.* Earl in the tech department who walks like he hasn't quite mastered the whole upright evolution thing, matched only by his choice of grunts over actual language? *Low vibe.* Putting science aside, we *know* this stuff. There are people who leave you feeling energized, empowered, and pumped up to be around. There are also people you have to mentally prepare to interact with, knowing that a ten-minute conversation with them can leave you feeling like you just ate some sweaty gym socks and are now trying to digest them and forget this encounter ever happened. That's not just a matter of enjoying one person's company while finding the other annoying. That's energy. That's their vibration, the energy they are putting out into the world.

And how do you think this plays out for them? Again, putting science aside, let's think about personal experience.

I used to work with this guy Greg. Greg's seemingly favorite expression was "of course." As in, "Damn it, *of course* it's raining on the one day I took my umbrella out of my car" or "Are you kidding me?! *Of course* they call a last-minute meeting on the day I have a raging migraine." From Greg's point of view, the world was out to get him. Anything that could possibly go wrong for him, would. *Of course.* It didn't matter the situation; Greg would find the negative:

Me: "Hey, check it out! Work got us catered lunch!"

Greg: "Ew. Of course, they got it from DiAngelo's. I hate that place."

Me: "No work on Friday, buddy! Loooong weekend, here we come!"

Greg: "Yeah, except that I have to be in super early Monday morning for a meeting, of course."

Me: "Hey man, how'd your date go last weekend?"

Greg: "Well, of course she was late, so the restaurant was packed by the time we got seated, leaving us to sit right by the bathroom."

There was just no winning with this dude. *Expecting* the negative came naturally to him, so, when it showed up, as it always will when you're searching that hard to find it, it just cemented his belief that he was destined to be the victim.

What kind of energy was Greg putting out? Personally, the kind I'd like to stay away from. In the wise words of rapper/songwriter Kendrick Lamar: "Bitch, don't kill my vibe."

Just like those tuning forks, Greg is constantly sending out low energy. Putting aside the fact that even if a big break did come his way, he wouldn't recognize it for what it was, in all likelihood it won't. Science has shown us that like attracts like. Greg will surround himself with similarly negative people who feed off each other's low-energy vibes. He'll continue to put himself in low-energy situations, because that's not only where he feels comfortable but also what he is attracting to himself.

On the other end of the spectrum is my friend Jadyn. *Holy mother of all optimists, Batman.* In Jadyn's world, everything is destined to work in her favor. I have personally watched this girl reap everything from free coffee to comped bar tabs, to being pulled onstage at nearly every event we've ever attended. It's become a running joke in our circle that if there's a prize to be won or a person to be chosen, it will be Jadyn. While Jadyn is very pretty, it's not a looks thing that makes her stand out. Jadyn puts forth this energy of "Isn't this fantastic?!" in every situation, from a simple night at the movies to a trip to the dentist.

It's not a fake bubbly personality. I've seen the girl go through her fair share of shit, and she cries and vents with the best of 'em. But her everyday approach to life is the polar opposite of Greg the Grump's "Life is out to get me" perspective. Hers is more like "Life is a party, and I'm here to get the crowd dancing!"

It's not a coincidence, then, that all this stuff seemingly falls in Jadyn's lap. She doesn't work harder than any of our other friends. She's not miles ahead when it comes to intelligence or looks. Everyone in our circle is about even on all those playing fields, given that like attracts like. Jadyn's *energy* sets her apart. It's what attracts positive things into her life. And when those positive things come in, she expresses gratitude, celebrates them, and keeps on livin' it up.

Good things coming in only raise her vibration higher, so they keep on comin'.

RAISE YOUR ENERGY

Our energy comes first and foremost from our mindset.

If you're living in Grumpy Greg's world and you've trained your mind to focus on and expect the worst, that will continue to be your default until you do the work to rewire that sucker. As we've seen, our thoughts are the birthplace of our feelings and actions. If Jadyn walked around having thoughts focused around how terrible everything is and feeling like the world is out to get her, I don't care if she's winning Golden Globes in her spare time, no amount of acting could cover up her energy.

Doing the mindset work in this book not only helps you to establish lifelong habits when it comes to health and fitness, but it will also raise your vibration. When you walk around knowing what a powerhouse you are, you put forth that confidence into the world. It's in how you walk, how you talk, the actions you take, and the vibes you put forth.

Your mindset also ties directly into your health, which is the second factor in raising your energy.

My absolute favorite part of working with people is watching their internal transformation. Because health and fitness transformations take time and consistency, the outward results don't appear as drastic right away from an onlooker's perspective.

*It's the image my clients hold of themselves that is the first to change, and **that's** what makes all the difference.*

When Joni and I first started working together, she told me:

> "I have three pairs of work pants that I rotate between. I hate how they look but they're a size too big, so I don't have to feel them digging into my stomach when I sit down."

> "I've just learned not to look at my reflection. I feel like shit about myself when I see it, so why put myself through that?"

> "I'm tired all the time. I want to make changes, but I just don't have the energy. I feel stuck. I'm beginning to feel hopeless."

Stuck. Hopeless. Constantly thinking about ways to avoid seeing yourself in mirrors. Talk about an energy suck. I don't care how much money you have in the bank, what kind of car you drive, or what vacation pics you're plastering all over social media, if these are the feelings you're having about yourself, there is simply no way you're living a high-vibe life. And it follows that you're attracting back more of the same.

If you want to raise your vibe, the literal vibrational waves you're putting out into this world, you must raise your energy. This means training your mindset *and* your body. Not to look a certain way or reach a specific goal weight, but for the *feeling* it gives you.

Within three weeks of working together, Joni had lost ten pounds. It was a good amount of weight, definitely worth celebrating. But given Joni's goals (she had about seventy-five more pounds to go), it wasn't enough for a passerby to notice a change. That meant absolutely nothing in Joni's world. This girl was *on fire*.

"Rachel," she would message me, "I feel ahhhhmazing. In fact,

I treated myself to a new pair of pants, ones that **actually fit**, to celebrate the work I've done in these past weeks."

She started taking progress pictures and posting them on social media. She started sharing her journey with her family and friends, inspiring others in her family to jump onboard. Her feelings of shame and discomfort were replaced with pride, excitement, and empowerment. Keep in mind, to most, she outwardly looked like the same person. The biggest change had nothing to do with those ten pounds she had lost. It was her mindset that had changed. She had invested in herself and knew she was on a path to change her life. She was high vibe for the first time in a long time.

Suddenly, seemingly random things started lining up for her.

Part of Joni's overeating was because she used food as comfort when she felt lonely. She lived alone, and usually found herself mindlessly snacking while watching late night movies. Her evening thoughts were often focused on the desire to have someone to share her home with, and food filled the void that she felt.

Once Joni identified that she was using food as a comfort when what she really wanted was a companion, she started making changes. She set up an online profile and soon met a guy she liked and started seriously dating.

Joni's former low-vibe attitude had also been affecting her performance at work. Previously, she spent most days filled with dread, sitting in her cubicle, snacking away mindlessly, with the only "relief" being yet another hour-long staff meeting where she felt like all eyes were on her, judging her weight. Now she practically pranced into the office, excited to update her coworkers on her progress, and munched happily away on her goal-aligned snacks. The result? She got promoted. Big time.

As Joni put higher vibrations out into the world, she attracted more of the same right back. Despite still having more weight loss to go, she felt like a new person, and that's who she showed up as in the world.

With consistent effort in putting out the energy she wanted to receive back, Joni completely unleashed her best life. She's now living with her long-term boyfriend, is ten pounds away from her goal weight, loves her job, and, most of all, loves the Joni that shows up every day.

This isn't about a goal weight or a certain way you need to look. Goals are a great way to keep us inspired. But there will never come a time where you say, "OK, I'm healthy enough now" and stop. Because by the time you hit that goal weight, the bar will be raised, gym pun totally intended. It's not about that one particular goal. It's about how you *feel*. And how you feel is the you that shows up in this world.

And the you that shows up in the world is matching the vibration of every single thing the world is sending right back to you.

SELFISH, NO. INVINCIBLE, YES.

I like to give Victoria credit for being the inspiration behind my company because she was the first to verbalize how feeling empowered was an even bigger deal outside of the gym than in it. But the full story is that it happened a bit more organically than that.

Once coworkers started seeing and hearing about the new badass

Victoria, a few others jumped onboard. Soon, we had our little prework morning gym crew. More feedback like Victoria's started rolling in:

> "I can't believe that, despite waking up at 4:45 a.m. to train at 5:30 a.m., then go teach all day, I have *drastically more* energy now than ever before!"

> "Know what I did this weekend? Put on a bathing suit! Me! In a bathing suit! I haven't worn anything but shorts and an oversized shirt since I had kids!"

> "I absolutely cannot believe that I miss the gym on the days I don't go. I never thought I'd be this person. I just feel so good after a workout that I crave it now!"

> Even: "I've had more sex with my husband this month than the past six combined! I haven't felt sexy in a long time and, man oh man, does it feel good!"

As with Victoria and Joni, these women didn't look drastically different on the outside yet. It was how they felt about themselves that had changed, and that was rolling over into every area of their life.

When I tell people this story, I often hear responses such as "That's amazing and I would *love* to experience that kind of transformation, but between work and my family, I just don't have time for myself."

This makes sense, especially for those of us who tend to be givers. People who are givers by nature tend to put themselves last. Any deviation from this "others-come-first" comfort zone and, well, we know by now how our caveman brain would feel about *that* shift.

You're a teacher. Your day starts with getting your kids, your spouse, and your dog ready to get out the door on time. Breakfast? What's that? You have enough on your hands making sure your kid is wearing pants.

You're greeted at the steps of the school by a parent who, surprise, surprise, arrived twenty minutes early for your conference and is now following you up to your classroom, explaining why their child deserves a chance for extra credit despite not having done a single homework assignment all year.

The bell rings, and your day begins, much of which is spent taking deep breaths, smiling, and reminding yourself that a ten-year-old is not expected to have the same cognitive function as an adult, so it really is OK that they asked a question for which the literal answer *just came out of your mouth.*

Lunch? Sure, if you enjoy trying to use a fork and copy machine at the same time while balancing a glass container containing cold leftovers because you don't have time to wait for the microwave since copies need to be made on the printer that was broken this morning when you had a whopping ten minutes reserved to make them.

School ends and it's staff meeting time. Don't worry, it'll just be an hour.

Two hours of listening to your boss read bullet points off of a PowerPoint presentation about something that easily could have been an email, and you're now racing home to get the kids before they're late for soccer practice yet again.

Soccer's over and it's time for dinner. What? You didn't cook? You better figure something out, and quick. The kids are getting hangry. But wait, you didn't finish tomorrow's lesson plans! You don't have time to cook! OK, fast food it is, but just this once.

As you pull in the drive-through for what's actually the third time this week, your daughter tells you her book report is due tomorrow, and you forgot to proofread it like you promised.

OK, proofread first, lesson plans second. But, wait. You promised your spouse you'd look at the potential houses he emailed you, because buying a new home is seriously what you need to add to your plate right now. But, alas, you promised.

OK, proofread, houses, lesson plans. Looks like you're in for a long night.

Eleven o'clock and you're finally laying down to sleep. You mentally calculate, *OK, if I fall asleep right now, I can still get six whole hours of sleep* over and over until you're down to four hours of sleep if you drift off right this minute.

Just as you feel sleep finally creeping in, you remember: *Ugh. Today was the day I was supposed to start my new gym routine.*

Teachers tend to be givers. Everyone else gets first priority, leaving their own health and happiness as a "When I Have Time" activity, which typically equates to never. This isn't only true of teachers, of course. Anyone who consistently puts their wants and needs on the back burner while they attend to those around them know this story all too well.

What's more, our society creates martyrs of this behavior:

"Oh, she's the sweetest! Such a giver!"

"That guy puts everyone else first. He's one of a kind!"

But there's a major issue with this:

The you that's showing up tired, run-down, and hanging on by a thread is not the best version of you. And it's definitely not what you want the people you love to emulate.

Kids are smart little suckers. They're picking up on a whole lot more than we tend to give them credit for. That fake smile doesn't override the fact that two minutes ago you momentarily snapped at little Joey for the light pencil tapping that sounded like a jackhammer to your sleep-deprived brain. All the stickers and glitter in the world won't make up for the fact that your energy in the front of that classroom is on par with last week's two-hour PowerPoint hell meeting.

Those little off the cuff remarks about how "there's never enough time" and "wake up, Sammy, we're all tired, but now's not the time to catch up on sleep" are being absorbed as life lessons by those kids. You're sending the message both verbally and energetically that being tired, worn-down, and hanging on by a thread is the norm in life, because that is your current reality.

It doesn't have to be that way, and you can show them that through example.

The you that's going through the motions with your spouse.

That unconsciously stiffens every time they touch you, in fear that they feel a jiggle somewhere on your body you don't want them to.

That knows you should be having more sex but, let's be honest, who has the energy at the end of the day anymore?

That settles into a routine to just survive until the weekend.

That tells yourself, *Everyone feels burned-out. I'm doing this for a good cause.*

That knows deep down this is not the life you dreamed of but has rationalized why it's good enough.

That's not the best version of you.

*That's not the you the people in your life deserve. And it's 100 percent not the you that **you** deserve.*

Taking care of yourself first is not selfish. It's the most important thing you can do for those you love.

When you take care of yourself both physically and mentally, you raise your own energy. Raising your own personal energy attracts more of that energy into your life, that same life that you share with your loved ones. They, in turn, not only get to reap the benefits of this new, empowered you but also that of the new, empowered life you are attracting. In turn, chances are *they* will start to make a shift as well. That part is up to them.

But *you* are up to *you*.

Life is energy. You attract back what you put out. If you want to live an empowered, badass life, you *must* begin by feeling like the badass you were meant to be, the badass you are. That means putting in the work to take care of *you*.

Selfish?

No.

It's the most powerful gift you can give to the world.

Put in the Work

Rate your *current* situation in each area from one to ten, openly and honestly. One would be "Low Vibe" while ten would be "High Vibe." No judgment here. As with everything else in life, step one is to get honest and shine the light of awareness on our current situation so we can then move forward.

- When I think and talk about my current weight, I feel:
- When I think and talk about my current relationship with food, I feel:
- When I look in a mirror or catch a glimpse of my reflection, I feel:
- When I think and talk about my energy level, I feel:
- When I think and talk about my daily schedule/time in a day, I feel:

Now let's look at the result of the vibes you're putting out there. Again, we're looking for 100 percent honesty. The purpose of this isn't to judge yourself. On the contrary, it's time to celebrate! We're taking the steps toward change, and that's a huge freakin' deal. Rate the following questions from one to ten, with one being "Unhealthy" and ten being "Fantastic."

- My relationship with my weight throughout my life thus far has been:
- My relationship with food throughout my life thus far has been:
- My self-talk about my physical appearance throughout my life thus far has been:
- The number of new, energetic, exciting adventures that have shown up in my life have been (one would be "None" and ten would be "Many"):
- I often have "me time." I find blocked off periods of time without disruptions to relax, unwind, and partake in activities that refresh me (one would be "Never" and ten would be "Always"):

Now's the time to take the filter off. Don't let that inner dialogue tell you what is or isn't possible. Just write.

- Imagine yourself at your goal weight. You've put in the work and it shows. Your clothes fit like a glove, and you're free to strut accordingly. Describe your vibe. How do you carry yourself? What's different about the you that's showing up every day? Write it down.
- What results would this version of you attract back into your life? Be specific. Health, physical looks, job, relationships, family, write it all down. Again, no filter, no need to be "realistic." Just write.
- Imagine yourself in a healthy relationship with food. You are 100 percent empowered with the tools to make healthy choices aligned with your goals the majority of the time while still allowing for the foods you love. You no longer guess as to what will work or what won't. You are in control, and you feel confident that you know how to achieve your goals using food as your fuel. What's different about the you that shows up every day? Think about both actions in a day *and* thoughts. Write it all down.
- What results would this version of you attract back into your life?
- You can't believe how smokin' hot you look! You can't wait to catch a glimpse of yourself in the mirror, as it's another opportunity to celebrate the work you've put in and the results you've achieved. You

can't believe this is actually you. What's different about the you that shows up every day? Think about both actions in a day *and* thoughts. No filtering.

- What results would this new, self-empowered version of you attract back into your life?
- You wake up every day before your alarm. You're upright and bolting out of bed, ready to rock 'n' roll with the day ahead. You feel amazing. Your energy level is through the roof. What's different about the you that shows up every day?
- What results would this new, high-energy version of you attract back into your life?
- You've worked out a plan that gives you nonnegotiable "me time." It includes a half hour every single day, and an afternoon block on the weekends. Your family is onboard, and you've all agreed nothing can come between you and your time. You can use it for bubble baths, a jog, getting your nails done, going to the gym, learning archery, anything and everything you've always dreamed of. What's different about the you that shows up every day?
- What results would this new, refreshed version of you attract back into your life?

CHAPTER VIII

FAT LOSS: CALORIES IN VS. CALORIES OUT

"If lovin' pancakes is wrong, I don't wanna be right."
—RACHEL FREIMAN (*SERIOUSLY, WHAT'S THE POINT IN WRITING A BOOK IF YOU CAN'T QUOTE YOURSELF?*)

If we want to start raising the vibration we put out into the world, we need to start by raising our physical energy.

Living a life where you constantly feel tired, worn-down, and uncomfortable in your skin isn't serving you. If you want to raise your vibe, it's time to make a change. This means no longer wasting energy on that unhealthy relationship with food. It means getting the body you've always dreamed of. Not only to *look* a certain way but, more importantly, to *feel* the way you want to feel. It means getting control of the fuel we put in our body: the calories we eat.

This starts with getting educated about the truth behind nutrition.

As a former teacher, the need to educate runs deep. Ask me a yes or no question and you will not get a simple one-word answer. I have a need to teach a person to fish, not give them a fish. While I'm sure this makes for annoying social situations (Seriously, can you imagine being at a bar and asking, "Is it bad to drink booze while on a diet?" and getting a complete nutritional dissertation in response?!), it's great news for you. Today's the day you learn the *truth* about nutrition.

The health and fitness industry is filled with more *do this and it will work* systems than would fit in this book:

- Point systems
- Frozen meals
- Wraps
- Pills
- Magic fairy dust

You name it, it's out there. Ask why it works, and you'll get an explanation of *how to follow the system*, not an actual scientific explanation of *why*.

There's a big difference between:

"Only eat fifteen points' worth of our food each day and you'll lose fat."

and

"Eating less calories than you burn in a day is mathematically and scientifically the only way to lose fat."

The first explains *how* to follow one particular system. The other explains *why* the system works.

So, you might think, *as long as it works, why do I care why?*

As we discussed in chapter 1, not knowing is not sustainable. When we blindly follow someone's system without getting educated as to how this weight loss process works, we're bound to that system. We are now stuck buying their frozen meals or only eating foods "allowed" by that program for, *gulp*, the rest of our lives.

Traveling? *Better find a place that carries their food.*

At a party? *Stay away from that buffet.*

Sick of their meals? *Well, suck it up, Buttercup.*

How many people do you know, and you might be including yourself here, who saw great results on a program, only to gain the weight back once they got off of it, simply because they had *no idea* why it worked and, by extension, *how* to keep it going without being on that exact program?

There was Karen in Accounting who drove everyone crazy with her insistence that Keto was The Holy Grail of Fat Loss. Until six months later when she regained all the weight she lost, plus an extra ten pounds.

And what about Uncle Jerry's famous Atkins Diet Extravaganza of 2007? He drove the family nuts with his dissertations on why bacon is the key to fat loss. Until he wound up in the hospital with a heart condition and strict orders to stop eating so much freakin' pork.

Lest we forget, there's also your personal Low Carb Cult of 2009, where you deemed carbs the root of all evil and lectured friend after friend about why going low carb is the answer to their weight loss woes. Until you cracked and ate your weight in linguini a month later.

We're here to break the cycle.

By learning how fat loss works according to math and science, not according to Fad Diet of the Month, we can do this once and for all as a sustainable lifestyle. There are hard and fast rules when it comes to fat loss and how the human body is designed that apply to all of us: you, me, Karen in Accounting, and Uncle Jerry. If you have a pulse, the rules apply.

Now, if at the end of this you decide, "You know what, Rachel? I understand that I can do this on my own. I get that I don't need to be reliant on any point system or frozen meals. But I want to. It works for me. I like it."

My answer, in the wise words of my former middle school students, is "Fantastic! Do you, Booboo."

My purpose is to educate you. To teach you the *truth* behind how fat loss works. To help you understand there's no magic to this, or even guesswork. It's math and science, and it works for everyone.

I want you to make an educated decision. I want you to know the truth. I want you to learn to fish. Metaphorically. I've only really fished once and I sliced my finger open, but that's a story for another day.

BREAK UP WITH YOUR DIET

Remember that relationship you stayed in *way* too long?

You bitched about it to your friends constantly. You told yourself repeatedly that *this* fight was the last straw. You fantasized about a new life outside of it. After each breakup, you swore you wouldn't go back.

And yet you did. Over and over again. You knew it wasn't what you wanted or deserved but convinced yourself that *this time would be different*. So, you tried again and again and again, only to experience the same feelings of unhappiness, unfulfillment, and frustration, again and again and again.

Until the day you didn't.

Ah, that glorious, freeing day when you decided *this is it*, and you *finally* left for good.

Yeah, it sucked at first. Big time. You had lost your sense of normalcy. You constantly questioned your decision. Your world was shaken.

But what happened? Within a few months, you looked back and thought, *What the hell took me so long?!* Once you saw it with clarity, you couldn't unsee it. You fully realized just how unhealthy that relationship had been and were left wondering why you didn't make this decision earlier.

Well, you're currently in an unhealthy relationship. You've been there your entire life, and, if you don't make some serious changes, you're destined to stay there for the rest of it.

This unhealthy relationship is with food.

If it helps, you're not alone. Most people will spend their entire sixty, seventy, eighty, ninety, one hundred years on this earth stuck in this unhealthy relationship and not even realize it.

*What the hell?! Karen in Accounting lost twenty pounds this month by cutting out carbs?! I've eaten nothing but salads for as long as I can remember, and I **gained** five pounds! That's **it**. No more carbs. Ever. Carbs are the devil. I REVOKE YOU, EVIL CARBS!*

*Ugh. Pasta bar day at work. What, are they trying to torture me? I've gone three days without carbs and now I have to resist **this**?! Well, maybe I should just have one little scoop of pasta salad. After all, I've been so good for the past three days. I deserve one little scoop.*

I can't believe I caved. I was crazy to think I could keep this going. Why would this time be any different? I'm just destined to be overweight my whole life. May as well go drown my sorrows in pasta.

Is this how you want to go through the rest of your life?

Because I promise you, unchecked, you will.

Fortunately, just like that ex you look back on and wonder, *What was I thinking?!* once you shine the light of awareness on this unhealthy relationship, there's no unseeing it. When it comes to nutrition, the answer, the key, the Prince or Princess Charming of this new life, comes from *getting educated.*

Taking the time to get educated about how nutrition *really* works is one of the most important decisions you will ever make for yourself. Once you understand how food literally fuels your body, you can begin to make choices aligned with your personal goals. That means no more living off willpower. Refer back to chapter II, Restriction, for a refresher as needed. No more cutting out entire food groups. No more "starting over" after eating a "bad food." Because, as you'll soon see, there are no "bad foods." It means eating guilt-free by making informed choices, not relying on a person or company to tell you what or when to eat, and living with crazy amounts of energy and a better mood consistently.

In short, *taking control of your health* and living like a badass all the damn time.

They say step one is admitting you have a problem. In our case, step one is acknowledging the unhealthy relationship you've been stuck in your entire life and *deciding it's time for a change.* To do so, we have to understand what's real in the world of nutrition and what's bullshit. We need to understand how nutrition works, not according to mass marketing, but true, nonnegotiable math and science.

We need to get educated, once and for all.

SPILLED COFFEE AND FAT LOSS

You wake up in the morning. You put on clothes. You brush your teeth (I hope). You walk your dog. You make a cup of coffee. You spill said cup of coffee. You make a second cup, in a travel mug this time. You walk to your car. You realize you forgot your keys. You walk back into the house. You mutter some curse words. You walk back to your car.

All of these activities burn calories.

Each day, you burn an average number of calories. Clearly this isn't an exact number. Some days you only forget your keys once. Some days you walk back to get them, get so distracted making sure your dog *really heard you* when you said that she's a good girl and Mommy loves her, that you walk back to your car only to discover you still didn't grab your keys, and the fun continues. More steps, more calories burned.

Nonetheless, it's an average. If your average day includes exercise, you burn more calories. If it doesn't, it includes less.

The average number of calories you burn in a day is called your *Total Daily Energy Expenditure* or *TDEE*.

This TDEE is the first key to fat loss.

Pause here and take a moment to look at your calendar.

What day is today?

Look at the clock.

What time is it?

Got it?

OK, mark it down because *this*, my friend, is the exact day and time you learn the secret to fat loss. The magic pill the health and fitness industry doesn't want you to know about. The key that unlocks every point system out there.

Ready?

Deep breath

If your caloric intake, meaning the number of calories you eat in a day, is *more than* your TDEE, you will gain weight. This is called a *caloric surplus*. If you figure out your TDEE to be 1,600 calories a day and you consistently eat 1,900 calories, you will gain weight.

If your caloric intake is *less than* your TDEE, you will lose weight. We call this being in a *caloric deficit*. If you figure out your TDEE to be 1,600 calories a day and you consistently eat 1,400 calories, you will lose weight.

If your caloric intake is *about even with* your TDEE, you will maintain, meaning stay where you are. We call this *maintenance*. If you figure out your TDEE to be 1,600 calories a day and you consistently eat 1,600 calories, your weight will stay approximately the same.

CONGRATULATIONS, GRADUATE! I hope you've enjoyed reading my book. *Goodnight!*

Just kidding, there's a lot more to this. But it really is this simple. As we know by now, simple doesn't mean easy. It means the concept is not complicated, despite what the health and fitness industry has led us to believe all these years.

So, the logical question is: how do you figure out your TDEE?

For those of you kickin' it old school, here's the formula to figure it out with quill and ink, or pen and paper, depending on your level of old school-ness.

If this seems daunting to you, not to worry. I have a free TDEE calculator just for your badass self on my website: www.MindStrongFitness.com/Becoming.

The first step to figuring out our TDEE is to get your BMR (Basal

Metabolic Rate), which is the number of calories required to keep your body functioning *at rest*.

Here's how you figure out your BMR:

FOR WOMEN

655
+ (4.35 × weight in pounds)
+ (4.7 × height in inches)
- (4.7 × age in years)

= **BMR**

FOR MEN

66
+ (6.23 × weight in pounds)
+ (12.7 × height in inches)
- (6.8 × age in years)

= **BMR**

So, if you are a 40 year-old-woman who weighs 150 pounds and is 5'4", your BMR calculation would look like this:

655
+ (4.35 × *150*)
+ (4.7 × *64*)
- (4.7 × *40*)

= **1420.30**

To get our TDEE, we need one more step,
to account for activity

If you are sedentary and don't exercise at all...
Multiply Your BMR by 1.2

If you exercise lightly* one to three times per week...
Multiply by 1.375

If you exercise to the point of really breaking a
sweat three to five days per week...
Multiply by 1.55

For intense exercise six or seven days per week...
Multiply by 1.725

So, if you are a 40 year-old-woman who weighs
150 pounds, is 5'4" and exercises one to three times
a week, your calculation would be:

1420.30 (BMR) × 1.375 = **1952.9**

---

which we would round to
1953 Calories
as your TDEE

---

*Light exercise can mean lifting weights that don't make you
grunt like a maniac or going for jogs that get your heart pumpin'.
It does not mean you powerwalk to McDonald's one to three
times a week. Also remember that the exercise descriptors for
your TDEE calculation are an *average*, so don't freak out over
the fact that you exercised three times last week but only once
this week. Choose the option that's *closest to your norm*.

Let's pause here for a note on exercise.

You may have heard the expression, "Fitness is 20 percent work-outs and 80 percent diet." The reason is in that formula above. As you can see, exercise is not necessary for fat loss. This is why nutrition is queen. If you do exercise, in addition to the cardio-vascular and musculature health benefits, you get to eat more food, as you're burning more calories. *Woohoo!* But if you don't exercise, you can still lose fat, because fat loss comes down to calories in versus calories out.

While any kind of exercise is good exercise, I am a fan of weight-lifting. Why? Because lifting heavy shit is fun. Also, while cardio is great for straight up burning calories, our bodies are designed so that the more lean muscle mass we have, the faster our metabolism runs. How do we build lean muscle mass? Lifting weights.

I like to think of it as money in a checking account versus money in an interest-bearing savings account. Cardio is cash in your checking account. It's great. You have the money. You can add to that money by working. But the cash that's in the account just sits there when you're not working. You have to be actively working to get more money in that checking account. An interest-bearing savings account, however, works for you all the time: when you're at work, when you're sleeping, when you're at the gym, when you're in the bathroom. Without any effort on your part, it's earn-ing interest, adding to the amount in that account, no matter if you're actively working in that moment or not.

Cardio burns calories when you're on the treadmill running. Weight training builds lean muscle mass, which speeds up your metabolism. This results in your body burning more calories throughout the day, even when you're not at the gym.

To be clear, lifting weights *does not* mean mindlessly swinging two-pound dumbbells up and down with one hand while you watch cooking shows on TV. It means pushing your muscles to do what they can't yet do. When you push your muscles to their max, you create tiny tears in the muscle fibers. It's less painful than it sounds, don't worry. When you rest, recover, and *fuel your body with food*, these tears repair and, *blammo!* Muscle growth. In other words, you have to lift heavy and consistently if you want those lean, sculpted arms or that booty that won't quit.

Oh, and that whole *getting bulky* thing? Shelve it in the Bullshit Aisle, along with point systems and frozen meals. *Lifting heavy doesn't make you bulky.* Your diet, the way you eat consistently, is responsible for the composition of your body. It comes down to whether you're in a caloric deficit (eating less calories than you burn each day), surplus (eating more than you burn each day), or maintaining. How you lift doesn't change. Your nutrition determines your body composition.

While a full discussion on weight training is outside the scope of this book, I have a plethora of resources to get you started in the gym. You can check them out on my website, www. MindStrongFitness.com/Becoming.

All that said, using what we're learning about TDEE and nutrition, you can do this without exercise if you choose to.

Nutrition is the most important component to fat loss.

So, let's get back to our TDEE and learn how it works. If you took the four minutes to use the formula above, *whoop whoop,* you're already on your way to a healthier relationship with food. Let's keep this going.

As we've discussed, the bottom-line truth to fat loss comes down to calories in versus calories out: eat more calories than you burn, you gain. Eat fewer, you lose. Stay even, you maintain.

This explains a few things:

1. It's scientifically impossible to lose fat and gain muscle at the same time. Don't shoot the messenger. I'll explain why.
2. Any system out there that works, whether it's a point system, frozen meals, or meal replacement, is putting you in a caloric deficit, eating fewer calories than you burn. It is the *only* way to lose fat. Period.
3. You don't need to cut out carbs, be in a low-fat diet, or repeat mantras while waving your hands over your burger to lose fat. You only need to be in a caloric deficit.

CHARMING FIXER-UPPERS AND OTHER BULLSHIT

I have a buddy, Aiden, who works in the real estate industry. When I was looking for my first house, Aiden and I were scrolling through properties online together and came across an adorable little house with only a handful of pictures posted on the listing.

"Aiden," I questioned, scrolling back and forth between the obviously Photoshopped bedroom and weirdly angled bathroom pics, "I can't tell if this place is super cute, really tiny, or both."

Aiden leaned over, ignoring the pictures I was still studying as intently as someone trying to find a nonexistent snack in the fridge despite having checked two minutes earlier, and read the description of the house.

"There," he answered, pointing to a line in the description. "That's your answer."

"Charming fixer-upper?" I questioned, trying to figure out how anything described as "charming" could be a negative thing. It's *charming*, for the love of God!

"Yup," Aiden replied, as if the answer were clear and this conversation was over.

Seeing the confused, or perhaps desperate, look on my face (I really wanted to like this house), Aiden explained, "In real estate terms, 'charming fixer-upper' is code for 'piece of crap.' It's small. It needs a lot of work. It'll probably be cheap...because it's a piece of crap. This is not your house, Rachel."

Aiden was right, of course. When I went to see the house, it was exactly as he said: small, in need of some serious TLC (more like CPR), and definitely not my house.

Every industry has its own set of "code words," those terms that one wouldn't *dare* to use around anyone else in the biz but get thrown around for marketing purposes to the general masses.

It's like when you work in retail and they tell you, "This offer is only good until Monday!" but every employee in the store knows a customer can get that price anytime if they only ask.

Here's the most popular one in the fitness world:

"Lose fat while you gain muscle!"

Let me be blunt here: when you come across a program promising that you will lose fat while you build muscle, run. Well, you already know how I feel about running. So, leave. Hang up on them. Delete the email. Scroll past the ad. Whatever.

If I could have one wish when it comes to health and fitness, it would be that we could lose fat while we build muscle. Or that donuts count as a health food. Call it a tie. But, alas, neither exist in our world. I know, I know. Don't shoot the messenger. This isn't Rachel's Laws of Health and Fitness; this is How Human Beings Are Designed 101. And, for better or worse, our bodies are not designed to build muscle and lose fat at the same time.

It is a physical impossibility for your body to be in a caloric deficit, eating fewer calories than you burn, and a caloric surplus, eating more than you burn, at the same time. It's like saying, "Tony's 6′11″ but also only 5′3″." What?! Mathematically, he can only be one or the other. It's a physical impossibility to be both. The same is true of your caloric intake. The number of calories you eat in a day is either at, above, or below your TDEE. To build new muscle, your body must be in a caloric surplus. It must have more calories than it uses to perform daily activities in order to build muscle.[11]

"But Rachel," you say, "The program I just spent a lot of money on *swears* they can help me build muscle while I lose fat!"

Well, let's look at this mathematically. Robin uses the formula above and figures out her TDEE to be approximately 1,600 calories a day. She's determined to build new muscle while shedding fat. Tell me: *should Robin be in a caloric surplus or a caloric deficit?*

We've already determined that she needs the surplus to build new muscle. A surplus would mean she's eating *above* her 1,600 calorie TDEE. But she'll need a caloric deficit to shed the fat. A deficit would mean she's eating *less than* her 1,600 calorie TDEE.

The answer is that *she can't do both at the same time!* Robin must decide what her goals are. Does she want to spend a few months building new muscle in a surplus then switch to a deficit to lose some fat and show off her new muscle, or would she rather shed the fat now and show off the muscle she currently has under there? Her answer will determine her daily caloric intake.

To say you can burn fat and build muscle means that your body can be in both a deficit and a surplus at the same time. As in the case of 6′11″/5′3″ Tony, um what?! It's a physical impossibility. In Robin's case, it would mean she's staying under 1,600 calories a day but also eating more than 1,600 calories a day. Again, *what?!* It doesn't make sense *because it's not physically possible.*

So here's your homework. The next time a company gives you their sales pitch of "Lose fat while you gain muscle!" ask them this: "If we can only build new muscle while in a caloric surplus and only lose fat while in a caloric deficit, how is it that your program defies the laws of math and science?" Then get their autograph and take a selfie because if they have cracked the code on defying these laws, they're destined to make Bill Gates and Warren Buffett look poorer than a college student with a Ramen noodle addiction. Until that selfie exists, the answer is simply *that's not how this works.* Our bodies are designed to do one or the other at any given time.

"Lose fat while you gain muscle" is the "charming fixer upper" of the fitness world. Now that you're in the know, don't fall for the sales pitch.

POINT SYSTEMS, WRAPS, AND SHAKES...OH MY

Eat fewer calories than you burn, and you lose fat. It seems too simple to be true, right?

> "But my cousin Sandra did this point system for six months and lost fifty pounds!"

> "My friend's aunt's brother twice removed only ate Paul's Prepackaged Meals for a month and lost fifteen pounds!"

> "Karen in Accounting replaced lunch and dinner with shakes and lost a tremendous amount of fat!"

My answer? "Awesome!"

All of the above can be true. The important part is *why*. Why do some point systems work? Why does eating only prepackaged meals sometimes get results? Why do some shakes and meal replacements work when done correctly?

The answer, drumroll please, is that in *all* of the above, the person in question is in a caloric deficit. Period. Any point system that works is taking your TDEE, putting you in a deficit, and then *assigning points to its food instead of calories.*

Instead of saying, "Your TDEE is 1,600 calories. With our system, Meals A and B are 400 calories each. Meal C is 600 calories. By eating only those three meals, you'll total 1,400 calories, resulting in a caloric deficit," the company is keeping you blind to the process and simply saying, "Meals A and B are two points, Meal C is six points. Eat ten points a day and you're golden."

Will it work? *Of course! It's putting you in a caloric deficit!* Will you be reliant on their food indefinitely with no idea why it's working or, even worse, how to do it yourself, so you're tied to that company and their food for the rest of your life? *Yup.* Is this something you can learn to do yourself without that reliance on a company or their system? *You bet your lifetime supply of frozen meals it is.*

And what about my friend's aunt's brother twice removed? He lost a ton of weight eating only preportioned food! Can you figure out why by now? He, too, was in a caloric deficit, eating fewer calories than he burned in a day. Just like that point system, companies assigning you a set number of snacks per day, using their preportioned food only, are simply replacing calorie counting with a spoon-feeding method (that's totally a snack pun) of what to eat and what not to eat.

"But wait, Rachel, this one's different! I have freedom! This one allows me to eat one 'free meal' a day!" Sorry, same rules apply. That free meal comes with a calorie range, does it not? The reason? Snacks + free meal within that specified calorie range = caloric deficit.

And what about Karen in Accounting's meal replacement shakes? You guessed it: caloric deficit. If Karen housed ten of those shakes a day without following the associated plan, which typically says to replace one or two meals a day with this chalky chocolate-flavored hell, she wouldn't see results. The only thing those shakes are doing is swapping out food calories in a normal meal for the (fewer) calories provided by her shake and, you guessed it, putting her in a deficit.

You can do it with frozen meals. You can do it with prepackaged snacks. You can do it with shakes or bars labeled as meal replacements. Or you can do it with real food that you love and enjoy.

At the end of the day, the *only* answer to fat loss is to get in a caloric deficit.

RELIANCE, RESTRICTION, AND ADAPTATION

So why am I such a big believer in understanding how to do this yourself, when these companies are seemingly doing the work for you? Why take the time to figure out your TDEE and learn to track your food if you can just sign on to someone's program and eat the food they tell you to eat?

Again, the "blind follow" sounds good in theory, *but it doesn't sustain us in application.*

Whether it's point systems, preportioned snacks, or meal replacement shakes, simply following someone's program without understanding why it's working results in you being reliant on that company indefinitely. The moment you stop using that company—because you can't afford it, because they go out of business, because you're traveling and their products aren't accessible, because you get sick of their food—you're right back where you started six months before: weight gained back, and frustrated, limiting beliefs about this not being for you cemented even deeper.

But wait, there's more!

Following these systems without understanding why they work isn't just dangerous from the perspective of being reliant on them. That's just the tip of the iceberg. In chapter II, we spoke about Restriction. We understand by now that our mind wants to do what we tell it not to. Well, imagine walking around in a world where nearly everything is off-limits except for the same few pre-packaged snacks that you've been eating for the past five months.

You're at a party and everyone around you is hitting up the taco bar. You glance over at the nacho cheesy paradise, sigh, and slowly make your way over to the microwave to heat up your frozen meal, the same one you had for dinner for the past four months. Even the dog feels bad for you.

You take your niece and nephew to their favorite pizza joint, where you can smell the freshly baked pies and handmade pasta dishes. As they chow down on slice after slice, you deny yourself one of the great pleasures of this world because heaven, I mean *pizza*, is not on your "approved food" list.

Can you feel the tension just reading that?

How long are you going to keep forcing yourself to do something you don't enjoy? A month? Three months? *Maybe* six months? Restriction does not and will not work long-term.

When we get educated, we empower ourselves to make choices aligned with our health and fitness goals. We understand not only how to do this but also why it's working, so we can eat the foods we love while still hitting our goals.

And we're not done there!

Besides reliance and restriction, there's a third issue with blindly following these types of programs. Most of these programs are set up for quick and drastic results. While this is great for a short-term fix that will last just long enough to make your ex eat their heart out at your upcoming reunion, *you're setting yourself up for failure*.

Our bodies are powerhouses at adaption. It's the reason you

found a new normal after that breakup you thought you'd never get over. It's the reason hearing people in California say *hella* isn't *quite* as weird anymore. It's also the reason these point systems can fuck up your long-term goals. We've all heard of the dreaded plateau when it comes to fat loss. You lose fifteen pounds the first month, ten pounds the second month, five pounds the third month, then a mere one pound your fourth month in. Our bodies adapt to lifestyle changes. Like postrelationship life, we find a new normal. If you went from eating 3,200 calories a day to 2,100 calories, the fat flew off at first. With time, however, 2,100 calories will become your new normal. Your body has adapted. So, you adjust and drop your deficit a bit lower as needed, and the fat loss continues. The issue is most of these point systems and prepackaged meal companies are relying on fast, dramatic results for advertising purposes. They want the six month before-and-after pictures that make you stop scrolling through your social media feed and click to see how you too can get such dramatic results.

What you don't see is what happens a year later, when you not only gain the weight back but also another fifteen pounds on top of it.

To get those fast, dramatic results, you had to get in such a low caloric deficit that there's nowhere else to go. Not only is that not sustainable long-term, as you *will* cave and binge eat if you're walking around starving all day, but it's also wildly unhealthy and unsafe.

In fact, many of the companies doing this advise clients *not* to work out during this time. Any guesses as to why that is? I'll give you a clue: ever try to work out early in the morning before you've eaten, and had to pause because weird-colored spots had taken over your vision? It's because you weren't fueled for your workout. Calories are literally the fuel of our body. If we're barely giving it enough calories to function throughout the day, any additional output, i.e., exercise, will cause us to pass out. It's like flooring the gas pedal on your car when the tank's empty. You're doing some serious damage to your body. Not exactly the picture of health and sustainability we're looking for.

The key to making this a lifestyle and staying consistent is in making it *sustainable*.

You don't need to starve yourself. You don't need restriction. You need to understand that fat loss comes down to calories in versus calories out and learn to apply this to your own life, all while eating the foods you love.

Which is exactly where we're headed.

CARBS, FAT, AND PASTA BABIES

It's a hard pill to swallow that fat loss is such a simple concept. We've been brainwashed to believe there's a quick-fix, magic diet out there and our lives are a frustrating scavenger hunt of trying to find it. Because the health and fitness industry is such a booming business, most of which is based on complicating a simple process and selling you products you don't need that promise instant results that won't happen, we push back against the simplicity of how it really works.

The fact that I've caught myself complaining about "what a pain it is" to input my address so groceries that I ordered *from my computer* can magically arrive at my door twenty minutes later, shows what an instant gratification society we live in. We would rather jump from fad to fad looking for that quick fix rather than accepting the truth that it really is as simple as calories in versus calories out *and time*. When we don't see instant results, we assume it's not working, so we quit and continue our scavenger hunt for the quick fix that we'll never find.

I promise you, there's no quick fix.

It really is as simple as understanding how to get yourself in a caloric deficit and staying there long enough to get results.

But I get it. This concept goes against what mass marketing has sold us our entire lives. In fact, I've found that people get more heated about attempting to prove this concept wrong than any other, especially in the world of social media. Well, trying to prove this concept is wrong is tied with people on social media insisting that I use steroids. I once got called a "douche canoe" for denying that I've ever used them. I'm not sure exactly what a douche canoe is, but it's definitely become a part of my daily vocabulary.

Nonetheless, when I have these conversations with skeptics online, the topic turns from point systems, prepackaged meals, and meal replacements, to carbs and fat.

"But Rachel, my sister's husband's best friend's wife lost twenty pounds by cutting out all carbs!"

"Karen in Accounting lost ten pounds in two weeks when she went on a low-fat diet!"

If cutting out carbs or being on a low-fat diet works for you, do it. But understand that it's not necessary or advisable. Our bodies are designed to process carbohydrates, fats, and protein. When you attempt to manipulate your body by cutting out an entire food group, you're messing with the system.

Now, I consider myself a fairly intelligent human being. I've also studied how the human body works enough to accept the fact that my powerhouse of a body does not need little ol' me trying to trick it into doing something it's not designed to do. That sucka is a complex system that we haven't even *begun* to fully understand. It works just fine on its own, thankyouverymuch. The barrier between us and health isn't that we haven't *tricked* our body enough. It's that we haven't yet taken the time to learn *how to give it what it needs according to the way it was designed*.

Which is exactly what we're here to do.

In the next chapter, we'll get deep into the health risks of attempting to trick your body by cutting out entire food groups. For now, let's keep it a bit simpler: it's a pretty terrible way to go through life. I don't know about you, but I freakin' love carbs. Not *oh, I really enjoy carbs*. Love. As in *would elope with and have little pasta babies with them if it were socially acceptable*. Take carbs away from me and I *will* turn into a raging bitch. Ever see someone completely lose their shit when asked if everything's OK because they seem a tiny bit on edge? Multiply that by a thousand and it begins to scratch the surface of how I behave on a low-carb diet. Besides my permanent carb-neglected-PMS-like-state, living in a low-carb world is the epitome of restriction. And you already know by now that restriction doesn't work long-term.

But let's put all logistics aside for a second. Let's assume that you: don't care about the long-term effects of cutting out an entire food group, and you have the willpower of a Navy Seal. So, you spend the next twenty years of your life attending various parties and never touching the snack table. You go to your best friend's bachelorette weekend and eat nothing but raw veggies (which are technically carbs, for the record). You go to your child's wedding and spend most of the night avoiding any area of the venue that could potentially put the cake within your line of sight. You attend your grandchild's Bar Mitzvah and eat nothing but plain gefilte fish.

Now you're ninety-nine years old and on your death bed. *What's important?* As you lie there and reflect on your life, do you really think your focus is going to be on how proud you are that you resisted carbs all those years? Or will you wish you had calmed the fuck down and eaten the damn cake?

The bottom line is this: not only is a life of cutting out carbs or fat not healthy or sustainable long-term, *it's not necessary.*

When it comes to nutrition, we're so conditioned to believe it's all in or all out. We've seen the hype that carbs or fat are the enemy, so we cut them out. Or we go the opposite route: we say "life is short, eat the cake" every moment of our life until we're fifty pounds overweight, struggling with low energy, and feeling like shit. How can we make a mindset shift once and for all? How about we break the pattern and develop a healthy relationship with food that *includes* the cake now and then, while eating for our goals the majority of the time?

When we understand that weight loss comes down to calories in versus calories out, there are no foods that are off-limits. There's no such thing as "good foods" and "bad foods." It's about making healthy choices aligned with our goals the majority of the time, while allowing for the foods that don't serve our goals as well every now and then. Taking control of our nutrition by getting educated empowers us. It changes our mindset from one of reliance on the next fad diet to one of freedom. It gives us choice because we understand *how* and *why* the process works. No more blindly following company after company or guessing as to what's working or not. We have knowledge and we understand Truth, and those give us power.

Because pasta babies have feelings, too.

Put in the Work

This chapter's work is simple. As you did when we started this journey with mindset, you're making a decision, a commitment, this time to get educated. You've already made the commitment to be "on," no more starting and stopping. Now let's make the decision to do this *once and for all*.

No more blindly following someone else's system.

If you decide later on that a system works for you, great. But you'll go into it with eyes wide open, understanding how it works and knowing that you have all the tools to fly solo whenever you choose. For now, commit to getting educated. Grab your journal and write out the following declaration:

"Today [date], I am breaking up with my diet, once and for all. No more jumping from fad to fad, searching for some nonexistent magic pill. Today, I commit to getting educated on how health and fitness truly work. It's time for me to empower myself and create a healthy relationship with food that will last for the rest of my life.

Signed, [your signature]"

CHAPTER IX

INTRO TO MACROS

"A life without pizza is a life half-lived."
—CONFUCIUS...*JUST KIDDING, STILL ME*

My old training buddy and best friend, Alex, had smoked a pack of cigarettes every single day for nearly ten years by the time we met.

Alex is what pop culture would call a Boss Ass Bitch. You name it, she's on it: runs her own business like a boss, owns her house and car like a boss, works out five days a week like a boss. She's basically walking song lyrics about a strong, independent woman.

Yet, try as she might, this Boss Ass Bitch seemingly could not kick her smoking habit. I watched her run the gamut of antismoking techniques: patches, gum, even hypnosis. To be honest, that one wasn't nearly as funny as I imagined it would be. No quacking duck noises involved. Bummer. Each attempt would stick for a few days, maybe a few weeks, then back to Old Smokey she went.

One night, we were having a cocktail or three with some mutual friends. Rejoining the group after her third smoke break that hour, the conversation turned to Alex's struggle with kicking the habit. One well-meaning-if-not-slightly-buzzed-and-no-idea-of-the-shithole-he-was-about-to-step-into friend commented, "Not smoking is simple. You just don't smoke."

The vibe in the air following that comment was a mix of nervous laughter and anticipatory held breath, as we waited to see if Alex would, in fact, lay this guy out on his ass in the middle of the slightly yuppy gastropub at which we were gathered.

Fortunately, Alex was on good behavior and the poor guy lived to see another day. But the thing is, he wasn't wrong. Not smoking is simple. You just don't light up. Yet Alex struggled to shake the habit. Why?

In our trip to the creepy farmhouse in chapter V, we learned that our brain literally gets wired for our habits, whether self-serving or self-destructive. Even if you're a Boss Ass Bitch like Alex, that ten-year, pack-a-day pathway is wired deep. Rewiring is absolutely possible, but it will take conscious effort, time, consistency, and a new plan. Leading up to that fateful day in the gastropub, Alex's autopilot was set on:

Eat: Smoke.

Stress: Smoke.

Celebrate: Smoke.

Booze: Smoke. A lot.

Left up to its own devices, her brain would continue on that ingrained path of least resistance indefinitely. It doesn't want to quit smoking! No more smoking means restriction. Restriction means discomfort. Discomfort means pain. And we already know that it's in our nature to avoid pain.

To quit smoking, Alex simply needs to stop putting cigarettes in her mouth and lighting them. To get there, however, Alex's best bet is to come up with a new plan: something to do instead of giving in to the craving, a new association of how to deal with stress or to celebrate, a new set of patterns, thoughts, and actions, taken deliberately and repeated over and over until they become her new, wired default.

The point is: saying something is *simple* is not the same as saying it's *easy*.

The *logistics* of not smoking are simple. Living a smoke-free life after a ten-year habit isn't necessarily easy. The same is true of fat loss. The *simple* truth is that fat loss comes down to calories in versus calories out. Is it *easy* to eat less calories in a day than you burn? That depends on how you go about it.

As we've seen by now, most of us have spent our lives attempting to achieve this goal of being in a caloric deficit:

- Not even knowing that was the goal. We followed someone's system without knowing why or how it was supposed to work.
- Having no idea how many calories are going in or out, leaving the process up to guesswork.
- By attempting to live a life of restriction or rely solely on will-power, which goes against our nature.

What we're learning is that the way to make this easier, and the way to make it sustainable, is by understanding how our bodies work, not according to mass marketing but according to math and science. In doing so, we learn how to balance the food we love, aka not living off restriction, in ways aligned with our goals. We understand why cutting out entire food groups is not only unnecessary, but unhealthy. We understand that there aren't any foods you "can't" eat. It's all about balance. Most of all, we get *educated* as to how this process works.

This isn't another "diet" in the "do-this-don't-do-that" sense. This is a lifestyle. It's a healthy relationship with food that you develop with practice and keep for the rest of your life. Once we understand how and why this works, it's simply a matter of repeating the process. We take the tools we learn here together and use them over and over until it becomes a wired pathway of how you not only eat on a daily basis but also how you view your relationship with food. The simple process becomes easy through the power of healthy habits.

TRUMPETS AND MACROS

Back when I was a musician, I used to invest a decent amount of cash in my instruments. They were, after all, how I made my living.

My first trumpet, purchased by my parents when I was in fourth grade, cost $450. It was a baseline student model, but it did the trick for what I needed to make my dying cow sounds as I learned to honk out "Hot Cross Buns." My student model trumpet had the three basic components: a mouthpiece (the thing you blow air into), the body (the main trumpet), and the valves (the buttons you push to change notes).

After four years of practice and considerable improvement, I had sufficiently proved my dedication to music, and my parents rewarded me with an upgraded, pro level trumpet. This one cost $1,500 and, boy oh boy, was it fancy! Silver plated, reverse tuning slide, and a name brand written right on the bell. I was livin' the band nerd life. Still, this trumpet had the same three components: a mouthpiece, the body, and the valves.

When I got to college and started freelancing professionally, I dug into my savings account for the first time in my life. My teacher had this *beautiful* copper-belled trumpet that I would drool over in our private lessons. I'd blame it on all the air I was blowing, but the drool was mostly from staring at the trumpet. Thirty-five hundred dollars later and an identical trumpet was mine. Although this one had that gorgeous copper bell, it still had the three basics: a mouthpiece, the body, and the valves.

No matter how fancy my instrument got, it always needed the basics: a mouthpiece, the body, and the valves. Take one of those three things away, and the instrument didn't function as it was designed. Yeah, I could make funny duck sounds on the mouthpiece alone, but it's not what it's ultimately designed to do. I *could* make a weird hollow sound on my trumpet without the valves in, but no one would pay to hear that. And, without the body, well, a trumpet is no longer a trumpet, and I'm out of gigs. To use the instrument the way it was designed, it needs all three components.

Your body is a beautiful instrument. Just kidding—this isn't a fairy dust and rainbows book, remember? But it does hold true that, just like my trumpet, your body is designed in such a way where it has specific needs to properly function. The needs, in the case of your nutrition, are where our calories come from. We call these calorie sources *macronutrients*, or, to sound less nerdy, *macros*.

When we refer to macros, we are talking about:

- Carbohydrates (carbs)
- Fats
- Protein
- Alcohol is also a macronutrient source, but it's beyond the scope of this conversation. (No offense, alcohol. Still love you.)

Check out the food label on anything you eat, and you'll find the carbs, fat, and protein—the macros—in each serving of that food. Each macro has a specific function, and all are necessary.

Before we get into the role of each macro and why we need each one, we need to understand the bottom line of nutrition. A common example when it comes to nutrition is your car. You can have the shiniest, fastest Lamborghini Diablo on the block, but if you don't put gas in it, it's now turned into a beautiful decorative piece for your driveway.

Like cars run on gas or electricity, our bodies run on calories.

Calories are literally our fuel. If you're living life with low energy, dis-ease (see where that word comes from?), digestive issues, and/or excessive weight, you are not broken. You are not a bust. You are simply fueling your body in a way it isn't designed to be fueled.

Cal·o·rie

/ˈkal(ə)rē/

noun

The energy needed to raise the temperature
of 1 kilogram of water by 1°C

Energy. Calories are measured in energy.

Before that can of SpaghettiOs hits your bowl, scientists had to figure out the calorie content. They needed to know what to put on that nutrition label so you could decide whether or not to use the calories (energy) in that food source as your fuel.

When I first learned how calories are calculated, it was a favorite tidbit of information to share. I'd tell people, "Calories are basically measured by blowing shit up!" While that may be an oversimplification, it stands that the process is way cooler than you might have imagined.

Calorie calculation is done with a device called a bomb calorimeter. Seriously, this is a real thing. Here's how it works:

> The food being measured, let's say a bagel, is placed into a vessel called a bomb. The bomb is filled with oxygen and placed inside a container surrounded by water. The bagel is then ignited by a current of electricity. The surrounding water absorbs the heat that is released as that bagel burns, baby, burns. The water's rise in temperature is then recorded. Since a calorie raises the temperature of 1 kilogram of water by 1 degree, the calorie count is found by

calculating the change in temperature of the water multiplied by the volume of water.

See?! Science is fun! You get to set food on fire!

So why the mini science lesson? Because understanding the importance of nutrition is a complete game changer.

When you grasp the concept that calories are *literally energy*, and the food you choose to eat is the carrier of that energy, we can begin to view food as the source of our fuel and make choices accordingly. With this knowledge, we can begin to understand that what we chow down on each day determines our health, our energy level, how our body functions, and how we feel each and every day.

KNITTING AND MACROS

It's time to dig deep into the world of nutrition. As we talk about each macronutrient, its role, and why excluding any one of them from your diet is going against how your body is designed to function, keep in mind that the word "diet" in this context is not the ol' restrictive diet we often associate with that word. Diet means how you eat in a day. My *diet* includes foods aligned with my goals the majority of the time, with the occasional Krispy Kreme and slice of pizza thrown in here and there. I am not *on a diet* that includes point systems and frozen meals. I *have a diet*, or way of eating, that I stick to consistently.

Once we're familiar with each macro, we'll go step-by-step into the process of what we call "macro tracking." *This* is where we learn to make nutrition a sustainable lifestyle. We'll see how much of each macro you're currently eating, determine how much of each macro is recommended as a starting point for your personal goals, and how to adjust so these numbers match up.

Here's the most important point to keep in mind: this is not Rachel's New Fad Diet or even Rachel's Laws of Nutrition.

I did not invent macronutrients or macro tracking. I have, however, found it to be the number one way to make eating for your goals sustainable. It's not based on restriction; you're picking and choosing what to eat and what not to eat, and there's room for virtually any food once you learn the process. Macro tracking is based on math and science. It works because it follows the laws of how our body is designed, in terms of processing all three macronutrients. It's also aligned with the psychological patterns of most humans, due to the shift away from restriction and the focus on choice.

It will take time and effort to learn. One of my favorite mantras for myself, my clients, and my former middle schoolers when they picked up an instrument or a new piece of music for the first time is: "Nothing in life is difficult; it's simply unfamiliar." Going into this with the mindset of learning a new skill that you'll have for the rest of your life, rather than the drudgery of attempting "yet another diet," will allow you to be patient with yourself and *fall in love with the process.*

When you decided to take up knitting, you could have focused on the first sweater you ever tried to make and gotten extremely frustrated, extremely fast: *Ugh. This sweater is taking forever! I could go to the mall and buy six sweaters by the time I finish the sleeve alone!* Or you can focus on the skill you're learning: *Wow! Knitting is intense! By the time I'm done learning how to make this sweater, I'll be able to knock out tons of other items! Christmas presents for everyone!*

The same holds true here.

If you've never tracked what you eat in a typical day, it's not realistic to expect yourself to flick a switch and start eating for your goals overnight. It will take time, practice, patience, and adjusting. Only you can decide if it's *Ugh. Tracking what I eat each day?! I could just eat the exact foods Freddy's Frozen Meals tells me to eat and be done with the damn thing!* or *Wow! This is incredibly eye opening! Seeing exactly what I eat in a day is helping me to understand not only how I got into the unhealthy situation I'm working to get out of, but it's also giving me complete power to take control of my nutrition. Once I get this skill under my belt, I don't need any company or program ever again. I will be in complete control of my nutrition! That's incredible!*

Like all of life, this process will come down to your mindset.

PASTA IS LIFE

Let's start with the macronutrient that gets the worst rap: carbohydrates (carbs).

There are three topics I've learned are better left untouched in polite conversation: politics, religion, and carbs. I've seen friendly chats go from, "Quite the weather we're having, eh?" to "HOW THE HELL COULD YOU EVEN PROPOSE SUCH ABSURDITY?!" at the mere suggestion that carbs do not inherently make you fat. We are living in a society that has deemed carbs the enemy and anyone who has managed to get in shape while eating this deemed culprit of obesity is labeled as a Freak of Nature.

Well, freaks unite! I'm here to shout it from the rooftops and set the record straight: carbs do not inherently make you fat. They are *necessary* for our body to perform at its best. Yes, you can quote me on that: *necessary to perform at its best.*

Before you go downing your weight in all-you-can-eat breadsticks, we need to understand that, while carbs themselves are not the issue, the *amount of carbs most of us currently eat* and *the sources of these carbs* are major factors in our current health woes. We need to understand *what kind of carbs* will best serve our goals and *how many carbs* would best fuel us so we can focus on those, while still allowing for those delicious, garlicky breadsticks. But first, we need to understand *why* carbs are so important.

BACON AND BANANAS

There are hard and true facts when it comes to health and fitness that remain intact, regardless of your personal preference.

For example, there's no denying that cardiovascular exercise improves lung function. The fact that I'd rather sit in the middle of a creepy butterfly garden, with those gross little legs crawling all over me and wings flapping everywhere, than step foot on a treadmill, doesn't negate the fact that cardiovascular exercise still improves lung function.

Carbs are our body's primary energy source. If you feel that your body works best without carbs or you choose not to eat them for religious reasons (I'm not sure what religion that is, but I'm assuming there's one out there), it doesn't discount the fact that our bodies were designed to go to carbs first for energy. Keep in mind that thinking your body works best without them very well may be because you've trained your body to function without them. This doesn't actually mean it's operating at its best, but rather that you need to readjust to how your body was *originally designed* before you thought you knew better than Mother Nature.

A quick rundown on energy in the body looks like this:

- Cellular respiration is a fancy way of saying *how we derive energy from the food that we eat*. Remember, calorie equals energy. We're literally breaking down our grub into useable energy.
- The majority of the food we eat in a day gets broken down into something called *glucose*, a simple sugar.
- Our body then breaks down this glucose to produce its cells' energy currency, called *adenosine triphosphate*, or ATP.
- Our body's *preferred go-to source* of energy is our friend carbohydrates, as carbs give us the most "bang for our buck" when it comes to easy ATP production.

Simply put, when your body needs energy, and it tends to need that a lot, it goes to carbs first.

Anytime we go on a low-carb or no-carb diet, we are *literally* attempting to trick our body to do something it wasn't designed to do. Will it adapt? *Yup.* Will it find a way to produce energy from other sources? *You bet.* Will you pay the price in the long run? *Of course.*

When you follow a very low or no carb diet, the goal is to put your body in what's called a state of ketosis. The idea is, *when you restrict the amount of carbs you're eating, the body will instead break down stored fat, creating molecules called ketones to use as fuel.*

The key word in that description was *instead*.

Your body *wants to go to carbs*. It is *designed to go to carbs*. It's only when it can't find those carbs that it makes other arrangements to produce energy. I don't know about you, but I don't want the backup plan. If I'm going in for major surgery and the receptionist tells me, "Our primary surgeon isn't here today, but we have our backup doc waiting for you. He's not the first choice, but he'll do." Um. This is my body. This is my health. Second choice won't cut it—especially in this case, when the first choice is there for the taking with a little education!

Listen, the human body is pretty freakin' impressive. Take one Intro to Biology class and your mind will be blown at the systems and processes in place that keep us alive as we sip on venti lattes with three extra vanilla pumps and binge watch reality TV. From breathing, to brain function, to energy production, there's an almost inconceivable amount going on in each millisecond of each day, and it's all happening without our conscious thought, guidance, or help. So, tell me:

*Why do we feel that the answer to getting healthy lies in **tricking** our body?*

If we have the confidence to trust our body to breathe without our help and keep our heart pumping without conscious thought, where along the line did we decide that our powerhouse of a body doesn't know how to process carbs, *the thing it was designed to go to first for energy*, so the solution must be to *trick it* into functioning another way?!

Not only do you not *need* to cut out carbs, but doing so is not healthy long-term.

We already know it's not sustainable as a "diet plan" due to its basis on restriction. What's more, studies are continuously coming forth on health defects of low-to-no-carb diets. The "keto flu,"[12] complete with fatigue, dizziness, nausea, and muscle soreness, often occurs because your body is no longer burning glucose for energy, which is its *natural way* to produce energy. Keto diarrhea (this is a real thing) is another common side effect,[13] occurring because your body can't keep up with processing such large amounts of fat in your diet. And, of course, there's the risk of heart disease when you're on a diet that calls bananas the devil but advocates for bacon![14] It's complete madness!

Repeat after me:

My body needs carbs to function at its highest capacity.

The problem, up until now, is not that you've been eating carbs. It's that you've been eating too much food in unhealthy proportions. Remember, fat loss comes down to calories in versus out.

The solution isn't to cut out all carbs. It's to get educated about how many you need, and which types will best serve your goals.

DONUTS FOR FAT LOSS

My middle school teaching years were filled with riveting conversations such as, "Who would win in a fight: Captain America or Hulk?" (Hulk, duh) and "Is Batman *really* a superhero or just a dude with a lot of money and cool toys?" The nutrition version of these hypothetical conversations translates to this:

> "OK, Rachel, so if fat loss comes down to calories in versus calories out, that means I can technically eat just enough Krispy Kremes to stay in a deficit and I'll lose fat."

In other words, "Is a carb a carb?" or "Is fifty grams of donut carbs the same as fifty grams of sweet potato carbs?"

The answer, to the surprise of many and the delight of most—OK, the delight of *me*—is yes. And no. When it comes to straight up fat loss, calories in versus calories out, a carb is a carb. Whether you eat fifty grams of Krispy Kreme carbs or fifty grams of plain old oven baked sweet potatoes carbs, you've eaten fifty grams of carbs. When it comes to *nutrition*, however, those fifty grams are extremely different.

What do I mean by nutrition?

Carbs, fats, and protein are our *macronutrients*, the calorie sources of every diet. We also have something called *micronutrients*, which are our vitamins and minerals. They're necessary for things like energy production, immune function, blood clotting, bone health, growth, and fluid balance. You know, kind of important stuff.

We need to understand that eating for fat loss does not necessarily equal eating nutritiously.

So, let's say your bestie, Kirsten, wanted to lose the three pounds she put on during your all-you-can-eat Alaskan cruise. Kirsten uses the information presented in chapter VIII and figures out her TDEE. Her goal is to lose fat, so she puts herself in a caloric deficit which, for her, comes out to 1,400 calories per day.

She could, in theory, eat all 1,400 of those calories eating donuts, pie, and ice cream, and still lose fat. A deficit is a deficit after all, and, when we're talking straight up fat loss, a deficit is all you need. The issue is Kirsten's body would shut down long before she could show off her new bikini bod that summer.

Donuts, pie, and ice cream contain very few micronutrients, or vitamins and minerals. Without these, our immune system goes to hell, our energy level goes *kaput*, and we open the door for a plethora of health issues. While the occasional slice of pie or ice cream sundae that fit into your daily calories won't hurt your progress, it's important to ensure you're making *nutritious* choices as we focus on our macros.

So, 1,400 calories from Krispy Kremes a day? Not recommended. Using up 190 calories of her 1,400 daily allowance for a Krispy Kreme every now and then while making healthy, micronutrient-filled choices the majority of the time? Not only will Kirsten continue to hit her goals, but she also has a significantly better chance of sticking to them, as she's *allowing room for her cravings* rather than attempting to live off of restriction.

Here's what that means when it comes to carbs.

There are two main types of carbs: simple carbs and complex carbs.

I like to think of simple carbs like a Tinder date: fun once in a while but, in general, not a lot of substance to them. Donuts, candy, syrup, cupcakes: all of these are simple carbs. The underlying theme of simple carbs is *sugar*. Whether processed or natural, sugar is broken down quickly. While this makes them great for a quick postworkout refuel, or a get-my-kid-jazzed-up-for-his-birthday-party-then-hand-him-to-my-spouse snack, it also means they won't keep you full very long because they're not very nutritionally dense.

Complex carbs are the Match.com to our Tinder simple carbs: more effort but also more fulfilling long-term. They come in the form of fiber and starch, are generally packed with more micronutrients—vitamins and minerals—than simple carbs, and they keep us full longer. Nuts, beans, whole grains, and vegetables all fall in the complex carb category. This is why large, nutrient-dense salads are such a great addition to your diet. Not only are you getting the vitamins and minerals packed into those complex carbs, but the fiber takes longer to break down, keeping you full longer.

Fruit is the awkward middle child between simple and complex carbs. While high in natural, unprocessed sugar, fruit is typically also high in fiber. This straddle between sugar/fiber/complex/simple is one of the reasons why fruit is such a hot topic of debate.

My opinion? Be honest: is cantaloupe the reason you're reading this book?

No? Then eat fruit.

The point of macros isn't for me to tell you what to eat and what not to eat. I don't know what you like, what you don't like, what you're allergic to, or what you're sick of eating. Remember, we're getting away from the "do-this-don't-do-that" mindset. I'm here to give you guidelines you can use to go forth and hit your goals *eating the foods you love.*

If you'd like some cheat sheets and reference guides on simple and complex carbs, you can grab them on my website: www.MindStrongFitness.com/Becoming. Keep in mind, these are *guides.* They are not "eat this, do not eat that" lists. We're learning information to get empowered, not blindly follow someone's rules of what to eat and what not to eat. We've seen where that leads too many times, and those days are over.

It's important to remember that, while a carb is a carb when it comes to fat loss, it will better serve your overall health and energy to make nutritious, complex carbs the majority of your carb intake. That said, and this is a biggie, *you do not need to eliminate all simple carbs from your diet!* While Rachel's Laws of Health and Fitness would clearly include a decree that "Krispy Kremes are hereby labeled a complex carb and should be eaten with every meal!" alas, that's not how this works. *However*, if a carb is a carb when it comes to calories in versus calories out, a Krispy Kreme factored in now and then *will not* undo your goals.

This is why I am such a believer that macros are the number one way to make nutrition a sustainable lifestyle. Your coach, the author of this book, someone who has done this and lived this, is flat-out telling you that the occasional donut is not only not off-limits but also *suggested* as a way to keep a healthy nonrestriction-based mindset. Making room on occasion for the foods you crave is a great way to ensure you don't go down the ol' restrict/binge eat path.

I don't know about you, but I was sold at donuts.

As we move on to the other two macronutrients, and head toward learning *how many* carbs to eat for your personal goals, understand that carbs are not the enemy. Carbs are important. They do not inherently make you fat. Your body goes to them first for energy.

And they're delicious.

We need to learn how to eat them in a way that's aligned with our goals, which is exactly where we're heading.

But first, let's move on to why a low-fat diet is literally messing with your head.

BRAIN FOG, FAT HEADS, AND AVOCADOS

One of the biggest struggles for me as a middle school teacher was not laughing at inappropriate things that kids said. From *yo momma* jokes to *that's what she said* comments, I often had to walk away so as not to break my poker face and crack up at jokes I actually found hysterical but was technically supposed to admonish.

As with the newest Air Jordans and jeans halfway off one's ass, the rip-on-your-bestie-topic-of-the-week came in trends. One of the weirder ones was around each other's hairlines. Yes, eleven-year-old boys would walk around teasing each other about their supposedly receding hairline. Considering I have yet to meet someone balding by the age of eleven, I never quite understood this one.

The other oddity was "Fat Head." Kids would tease their friends for having a head that was either too large or too small to fit the snapback they weren't supposed to be wearing in school anyway. Oh, kids.

The funny thing with Fat Head, besides the fact that it just seems like an odd choice of things to tease your friends about, is that, technically, we all have Fat Heads. Or, rather, fat brains. The human brain is nearly 60 percent fat.[15]

If you've ever attempted to go on a low-fat diet for a prolonged amount of time, you've probably noticed a few things:

1. It's not sustainable because, um, restriction.

2. Your brain feels foggy.[16]
3. Your hormones feel out of whack.
4. You get sick a lot more often.
5. It's not sustainable. Oh, did I say that already?

In addition to being an energy source within the body, fat is a carrier for certain vitamins and supports their absorption in the intestine. In other words, if the body isn't getting enough fat, you're not reaping the benefits of all those nutritious foods you're eating. When you're not getting adequate amounts of vitamins, your immune system isn't operating at full capacity and you get sick. Like, constantly.

We also need fat to build cell membranes and protective myelin sheaths (remember those from chapter V?).[17] Take away fat and bring on the foggy brain! Suddenly those cemented pathways that myelin did such a fantastic job of coating for us are a jackhammered mess, less like the smooth, cemented path to our farmhouse and more like the cracked, uneven sidewalks of New York City I used to constantly trip on. A brain composed of 60 percent fat needs the good stuff to operate.

Healthy fats help you feel fuller longer, balance blood sugar, and help to regulate hormones. Take away those good ol' healthy fats and *hellllooooooo*, hormone imbalance. (*Goooodbyyyeeeeee*, social life.)

Like carbs, though, fat gets a bad rap. We've been brainwashed (60 percent fat-brainwashed) into believing eating fat makes us fat. That's not how this works. Eating in a caloric surplus, eating more calories than you burn in a day, is what makes you fat. Eating healthy fats in proper proportions keeps your body performing in tip-top shape.

While a conversation on what makes a fat healthy or unhealthy is beyond the scope of this book, we can start from a place of logic: french fries, margarine, and donuts (sob) are all not-so-healthy fats. That doesn't mean we *never* eat them. It means we include them in moderation. Avocados, olive oil, and almonds are healthier fats. That doesn't mean we attempt to eat our body weight in almonds each day. It means they're healthier go-to options. For a list of suggested healthy fats, visit my website: www.MindStrongFitness.com/Becoming.

Your body needs healthy fats to operate at its best. The answer to achieving your goals doesn't lie in a low-fat diet. It's in choosing healthier fats the majority of the time, in the correct proportions for your goals, while still allowing for the occasional side of fries.

So, the next time a middle schooler calls you a Fat Head, tell them you hope they're one too, for health purposes.

Or make fun of their hairline. Whatever.

LEGO CASTLES AND MUSCLES

Back in my beginner weight training days, when both my gym knowledge and nutrition were a mess, I would spend hours in the gym working my ass off (or, more accurately, trying to build one) but not seeing much in terms of results. It was more than frustrating; it was deflating. What was the point in putting in all this time and energy if nothing was happening to my body?

The issue was, besides being low in carbs and fat, I also had very little protein in my diet.

Attempting to build muscle with insufficient protein is like building a Lego castle without the blocks. You're missing the component needed for the actual building. In other words, more than a minor detail.

Protein is the only macronutrient group that not only hasn't gotten a bad rap, but, on the contrary, has even become a borderline buzzword. From peanut butter to granola bars, it's hard to walk through the grocery aisle without seeing a food marketed as a "great source of protein." Companies like to throw around the term *protein packed* like it's glitter at a seven-year-old's birthday party. In reality, a lot of the food being labeled as such is not an actual source of protein, but a fat or carb source *with **some** protein in it.*

To start, let's talk about what protein is and isn't.

Despite what the packaging on many protein powders would like you to believe, eating or drinking protein alone will not give you big muscles. This isn't like Popeye downing that can of spinach and immediately bulking up. But, like Popeye and his can o' greens, you can't build muscle without protein. Believe me, I tried.

Protein is made up of amino acids. When you lift weights, you create tiny microtears in your muscles. When you eat protein, your body breaks it down and uses those amino acids to repair the tears. It's during this tear repair (say that ten times fast) that our muscles grow. No protein, no repair, no gunzzz. Protein is also an important building block of bones, cartilage, skin, and blood. You know, stuff that's pretty important.

Protein is also the one macronutrient that most people *aren't getting enough of*. When most people start paying attention to their macros, they're shocked to see their tendencies. While everyone is different, the common trend is to be high in fat and/or carbs and *low in protein.* Whether or not you're in the gym, but *especially* if you are, you need to ensure you're giving your body what it needs to build strong bones and muscles. Along with carbs and fats, that means sufficient protein.

If you're having trouble getting enough protein from whole foods, you can add in a protein powder. Note that *protein powders* are a *supplement* and do exactly what their name states: supplement, or *add to,* your diet. The goal is to get as much protein as possible from the foods you eat on a daily basis. If you're still not hitting your protein goals, a good protein powder can help you add extra protein in your diet. Like most supplements, there's a lot of crap on the market, so choose wisely. Along with a list of protein sources on my website, I've also provided a list of protein supplements I personally use and love: www.MindStrongFitness.com/Becoming.

Your body needs protein to build. Getting that protein from a variety of sources will ensure you're giving it everything it needs to function as it's designed to.

TRACKING: WHERE TO START

While a whole book can be written, and many have been, about the role of each macronutrient, it's not necessary to get started and make changes. What's important to understand is that we need all three macronutrients. If we're to go about our health and fitness goals in a way that's aligned with how our bodies are designed, that means including protein, fat, and, yes, carbs.

Eating any of these three macronutrients is not the reason you've struggled with weight loss. Eating too many of one or more of them is.

Right now, most of us can't even begin to guess how many grams of carbs, fat, or protein we're eating in a day. Not to worry! It's a simple and, in this case, easy process to figure out. If you check out the nutrition label on any food, you'll see a whole bunch of information. From Vitamin A to words you can barely pronounce, it's all there. Along with this smorgasbord of information, you'll find the carbs, fat, and protein content. In other words, that food's macronutrient content.

First and foremost, we need to look at the serving size on whatever we're eating. Sadly, and here's where I wish it were Rachel's Laws of Health and Fitness once again, an entire jar of peanut butter is not one serving. Two tablespoons are. The nutrition label on the average jar of peanut butter shows the following macros per two tablespoon serving:

Fat: 16 grams
Carbs: 6 grams
Protein: 8 grams

When we "track our food," we're recording the macronutrients of each food we eat. By the end of the day, we'll then be able to see how many grams of carbs, fat, and protein we've eaten that day by totaling up the macros for each food we ate.

Back when I was younger, along with climbing two miles uphill in the snow, we had to track macros by hand. Meaning, while my fingers were still sticky from that peanut butter, I was grabbing a pen and paper to jot down:

Peanut Butter:
1 (delicious) serving = 2 tablespoons
Fat: 16 grams

Carbs: 6 grams

Protein: 8 grams

And repeating the process for every food I ate that day, tallying up totals as I went. It's amazing I had any kind of social life with the time commitment this took.

A basic lunch alone would look something like this:

Peanut Butter:

1 serving = 2 tablespoons

Fat: 16 grams

Carbs: 6 grams

Protein: 8 grams

Whole Wheat Bread:

Serving = 2 slices

Fat: 2 grams

Carbs: 24 grams

Protein: 6 grams

Total for lunch:

Fat: 18 grams

Carbs: 30 grams

Protein: 14 grams

Fortunately for you, we live in the age of technology. Not only do apps exist to do the job for you, *free* apps exist to do the job for you! Nowadays (I feel like terms such as *nowadays* follow any uphill in the snow story), when you use an app to track macros, all you have to do is search the database for "peanut butter," adjust the serving to reflect how much you ate, and, poof, in your app "diary" go the macros. The app will show you lists, pie graphs, and bar graphs of the total grams of each macro you've eaten from the food you input, doing the math for you along the way.

Before we even think about how much of each macronutrient we need to eat each day, the first step to this process is to track our food. Why? When athletes want to improve their game, the first thing they do is watch videos of themselves in action. They study their current game footage for hours on end before taking a single step toward a new approach.

We must first shine the light of awareness on patterns and tendencies before we can make true, lasting change.

Just like those limiting beliefs we dug up, we have to first know what's really going on before we can do the work to make changes. This is 100 percent what tracking macros does for us.

I feel like I'm eating healthy/less/more aligned with my goals turns into *Here's **exactly** what I'm eating, so I know it's working. It has to. It's math and science.*

No more guessing. No more hoping. No more jumping from one method to the next. Macro tracking gives us hard, undeniable facts and, most importantly, a plan to hit our goals that's *not based on restriction.*

Today, we start with the first step: *tracking our food.*

Put in the Work

Today's work is a bit more logistical than what we've done so far. It can also be *extremely* eye opening when you commit yourself to it. This is where our mindset tools come to our rescue! If that caveman brain is telling you, *I can't do this* or *I'll never stick with this*, remind yourself that's Fear talking, talk to yourself like a kindergartener, and *keep going*. You've got this.

1. Download a free macro tracking app. I have a list of suggested apps on my website: www.MindStrongFitness.com/Becoming.
2. For the next five days, input everything you eat. Search the app's database of food and input the serving size you're eating. In the rare case that a food isn't listed in the database, most apps now have a function where you can scan the food to add it.
3. Don't try to make massive overhauls or suddenly start eating "clean." Just eat as you normally would and track, track, track.
4. You don't need to track water or exercise, just food.
5. Measure! When you input a food, it's going to ask how much of it you're eating. Guessing here will lead to wild inaccuracies. It's the difference between "I saved fifteen dollars yesterday" and "I saved a few bucks." Guesswork won't help us know where you are or where you need to go. Use measuring cups, measuring spoons, and a food scale. They take forty-five seconds of effort to implement and make a world of difference.
6. Commit yourself to five days of consistent tracking. No judgment. Just see the facts as they come and keep tracking.

CHAPTER X

MACRO BREAKDOWN

> *"Learn the rules like a pro so you can break them like an artist."*
>
> —PABLO PICASSO

WHOLE FOOD FRUSTRATION

I had a client, Adrianna, who came to me with the same frustration that many of us have felt when it comes to nutrition.

> "I just don't get it. I don't eat a lot of sugar. I gave up dairy. I eat fruits and vegetables. I don't eat a lot of fast food. I feel like I eat pretty healthy, yet I still can't lose these extra fifteen pounds. I feel like they're just stuck, no matter what I do!"

Adri's frustration was so intense, I wanted to hug her through the computer. She wasn't lying. She *was* eating healthy most of the time. She *had* made some important swaps in her diet when it came to overall nutrition. She *did* cut out a lot of junk food.

And, she was still eating more calories than she burned in a day.

About 99.999999 percent of the time, with the exception of a rare medical condition diagnosed by a doctor, the answer is always the same. Yes, you're eating healthier. Yes, you're making more nutritious choices. Yes, those things are fantastic for your overall health. And you're still eating more calories than you burn each day. You're going over your TDEE, that average number of calories you burn in a day, and the *only way to lose fat* is to stay under it.

If you're feeling a whole lot like Adrianna, today's your lucky day. It's the day you learn to fuel your body for your personal goals. Learning to eat according to the laws of how our bodies are designed is how you make this a sustainable lifestyle. No more guesswork. Total empowerment.

Let's learn how.

YEAH, BUT...

Before we jump into the how-tos of your macro breakdown, I want to put some common concerns at ease:

TRACKING EVERYTHING I EAT?! ISN'T THAT A BIT OBSESSIVE?!

Let's say you set a goal to save $10,000. The first thing your financial advisor is going to ask is "How much money are you currently bringing in?" followed closely by the next logical question, "How much money is going out?"

Responding with "I have no idea" gives you a pretty clear idea of step one: find out the hard facts.

Even responding with "I *think* I earn about $5,000 a month and maybeeee spend abbbbout $5,200 a month" will lead to the same step one.

If your goal is to save, we can't use guesswork. We need hard facts. Why? Because little expenses, such as a few bucks a day on lattes, can add up to huge dents in our current financial situation. Because bills on autopay that we set and forget still count toward our expenses. Because if we want to make a change, we have to know our actual starting point, not our best guess, which is often shockingly inaccurate.

Macro tracking isn't intended to make you obsess about every single calorie, but rather to put the hard facts on paper, or, in most cases, an app. It shows you *exactly* what's coming in each day in terms of calories. Like those lattes, it's often the small snacking that's the culprit. Other times, it's not knowing exactly what's in that morning egg white sandwich that was listed under the "lighter side" menu. Sometimes it's simply not realizing just how much we're eating at each meal or forgetting to account for that third glass of wine with dinner.

Macro tracking leaves no guesswork, just the facts. And that's the most important first step for change.

I PREFER TO EAT INTUITIVELY. I'LL JUST LISTEN TO MY BODY.

If you've trained your body to believe every Tuesday is Dollar Menu day, guess what it's gearing up for by Monday night? If you've taught it that 8:00 p.m. equals couch time and ice cream, you and Pavlov have something in common. Just like that bell signaling it's time to eat, your clock is telling your body it's time for cookies 'n' cream. If ten years of struggling to resist carbs has trained your body to reject them, that indigestion from sweet potatoes that you've accepted as "proof" that carbs are evil is holding you back from the sweet, sweet heaven that is baked sweet potato fries.

Right now, most of us have trained our body to have some seriously unhealthy daily habits when it comes to nutrition. "Listening" to it is not listening to its true nature but listening to it regurgitate back these unhealthy habits we've developed.

Eating intuitively, listening to what your body is telling you in regard to when and what to eat, is a fantastic goal to work toward. In fact, a lot of people use macro tracking as a tool to *get to* the intuitive eating stage. Once we fully understand how much we're eating in a day, what's in our common go-to foods, and how to "budget" for food not aligned with our goals, we're set up with the tools to do this with more freedom.

As Picasso said, "Learn the rules like a pro so you can break them like an artist." First, we have to learn and—wait for it—fully digest what's in our food. Then, we can use this understanding to make choices without being as meticulous with tracking.

I DON'T HAVE TIME TO TRACK MY FOOD.

Here's where we throw a little #biggerlifestatement into the mix. Change the words "I don't have time" to "it's not a big enough priority" and see how it feels:

It's not a big enough priority for me to track my food.

There's the truth.

We have time for what we make time for. Taking four minutes

to record a meal into an app won't become the focus of your Wednesday afternoon. You can find the four minutes while you're watching kitten videos on the internet. You can track it while you're in the bathroom. You can even preplan and track it the night before while you're eating your 8:00 p.m. portioned-out ice cream that now fits your macros.

When you decide you're serious about change, you'll make it a priority. And when it becomes a priority, you'll find the time.

This works when you do the work.

BREAKIN' DOWN THE MACRO BREAKDOWN: TOTAL CALORIES

Now's when we dig a little deeper and get a bit technical. Stay with me here and keep using your mindset tools. When that little voice starts to tell you, *This is too complicated* or *I'm never going to stick with this*, recognize it for what it is—your caveman brain equating change with death. Talk to yourself like a kindergartener, put your faith in me if it helps, and *keep going*. We're in this together every step of the way. Once you get the hang of it, these tools will empower you for life. It's worth a few minutes of math, I promise.

We now know that your TDEE, Total Daily Energy Expenditure, is your baseline zero. It's the average number of calories you burn in a day. Stay above it, you gain weight. Stay below it, you lose. Stay about even, you maintain. So, if your *only* goal is fat loss or gain, then the only number you technically need is your TDEE. But that's like saying, "The only thing I want in life is a ton of money in the bank." Is that really all you want? You don't want to spend the money? You don't want the feeling that buying nice things or presents for loved ones will bring? Is it true that all you really want is a lot of zeros on a computer screen?

We don't *just* want to see a certain number on a scale. We want to *feel* a certain way. We want to *look* a certain way. We want *energy*. We want overall *health* and *vitality*. To have all of this, we must take our TDEE one step further and discuss our macronutrient breakdown.

We've already discussed *why* including all three macronutrients is so important. Now it's time to learn *how* we ensure we're getting the right proportions for our body.

I want to be clear that this is a starting point. Like most topics in the health and fitness world, you'll find thousands of different viewpoints, all swearing they hold the truth on how to calculate macros. I'm here to provide you with some guidelines to use to get you going into the world of macros. As a starting place that's both personal and will work for everyone, we'll use these three steps below to find your macros:

1. Find your TDEE
2. Put yourself in a caloric deficit or surplus, depending on your goals
3. Break that number down into carbs, fats, and protein—your macros

The Put in the Work section at the end of this chapter will walk you through the process step-by-step to figure out your personal macros. For now, let's look at how this works.

You already found your TDEE in chapter VIII. Using that number, a good rule of thumb is to subtract 10–20 percent if your goal is to lose fat. This number is not set in stone, and it will change over time. This is a starting point. As you decide between the 10-20 percent range, keep in mind, as a general rule, you should never go below ten times your body weight. So, if you currently weight 130 pounds, your calories should never be below 1,300 (130 × 10). I suggest starting with a 10-15 percent deficit to let your body adjust, knowing you can increase with time, but you can be more aggressive with 20 percent if you feel it's sustainable.

For example, say you used the formula in the previous chapter and found your TDEE to be 1,900 calories. Your goal is to lose weight, aka be in a caloric deficit, so you would subtract anywhere from 190-380 calories (10-20 percent of 1,900), resulting in a daily caloric intake of 1,520 calories to 1,710 calories.

Keep in mind that *sustainability* is the most important factor here. If you subtract 10 percent from your TDEE and the number you get makes you want to cry, start with 5 percent. Hell, start with maintaining (you'll learn how below) until you get used to the process and *then* start subtracting calories to put yourself in a deficit! If you look back at the days you tracked in chapter IX, you can check the average number of calories you tend to eat in a day. That number may be much higher than your TDEE, so subtracting a hundred calories from that average could be a realistic starting place for you. The point is slow progress is *always* better than no progress. Being super aggressive with weight loss means nothing if it's not sustainable and done in a way that's setting you up to cave and binge. That tortoise knew what's up: slow and steady always wins.

If your goal is to put on weight, adding about 10–15 percent to your TDEE is a good place to start. Again, this will change with time, especially if you're in the gym and lifting heavy. This is a starting point. Say you used the formula from the last chapter and found your TDEE to be 1,900 calories. Your goal is to gain weight, aka being in a caloric surplus, so you would add 190–285 calories (10–15 percent of 1,900) and eat anywhere from 2,090–2,185 calories per day. If you don't mind gaining a whole bunch of weight, you can always choose to go higher in a surplus.

If your goal is to maintain, stay more or less where you are, your total calories will be the same as your TDEE, meaning, in this case, you would eat approximately 1,900 calories each day.

BREAKIN' DOWN THE MACRO BREAKDOWN: YOUR MACROS

Now that we have our total number, we need to divide this into our macros, our number of grams of carbs, fat, and protein we'll aim to eat each day. Remember that, for now, we're just learning how this works. We're going to walk through your personal numbers together, step-by-step, in the Put in the Work section.

As a starting point, I suggest using the following guidelines.

FOR PROTEIN, CALCULATE .8–1 GRAM PER BODY WEIGHT POUND.

If you weigh 130 pounds, your protein intake will be between 104–130 grams (130 × .8 to 130 × 1).

If you're actively working out, lean toward 1 gram. If you're not, stick with .8. Looking at your averages from your five days of tracking will also help. If you're currently only eating 40 grams of protein per day, jumping up to 130 grams might not be a reasonable goal yet. In that case, start with 104 and slowly increase. Again, macros are never "one and done." They require adjusting as you lose or gain weight and get closer to your goals.

FOR YOUR FAT, CALCULATE .35–.45 TIMES YOUR BODY WEIGHT.

If you weigh 130 pounds, this would put your fat between 46 (45.5) grams and 59 (58.5) grams (130 × .35 to 130 × .45).

If you want a few extra fat grams, go the higher route within the .35–.45 range. If you prefer less fat, leaving more room for carbs, as we'll see next, go for .35. All three macros will wind up equaling your total calories, so switching a few fat grams for carbs won't affect your fat loss/gain/maintenance goals. Remember, you now know that eating fat doesn't make you fat.

When working one-on-one with clients, I tend to give them more carbs than fat. As you'll remember, carbs are our fuel, so more healthy, complex carbs equal more energy. That said, macros are all about setting realistic goals that work for you, your lifestyle, and your preference. If you know you prefer more fat than carbs in your diet, lean toward the higher .45 option above, and, don't forget, you can always tweak later.

WHATEVER'S LEFT GOES TO YOUR CARB GRAMS.

To understand what "whatever's left" means, we need to do some nerdy nutrition math:

> One gram of carbs equals four calories.
> One gram of protein equals four calories.
> One gram of fat equals nine calories.

Let's say Casey's TDEE is 1,700 calories. Her goal is to lose fat, so she subtracts 15 percent from that number, putting her total daily calories at 1,445. Casey understands that sustainability is key, so she takes a moment to see if that number feels scary to her. Having weighed her options, Casey decides she's good with her 15 percent deficit and moves on.

Casey weighs 130 pounds and doesn't currently work out. So far, her macros look like this:

Protein: 104 grams (130 x .8)

Fat: 46 grams (130 x .35)

Since one gram of protein equals 4 calories, she's currently "spending" 416 calories on protein (104 grams of protein × 4 calories per gram).

Since one gram of fat equals 9 calories, she's currently "spending" 414 calories on fat (46 grams × 9 calories per gram).

When she adds her 416 carb calories to her 414 fat calories, we see that she's "spent" 830 calories so far.

Casey's total calories is currently set at 1,445. When she subtracts 1445 – 830, she's left with 615 calories.

Since 1 gram of carbs equals 4 calories, she divides those 615 calories by 4, giving her 154 (153.75) grams of carbs.

Now Casey's macros look like this:

Total Calories: 1446
(I've added an extra calorie so our nerdy math is exact)

Protein: 104 grams

Fat: 46 grams

Carbs: 154 grams

From here, Casey would input the above numbers into her app, and the game begins! Casey can eat the foods she loves, in whatever portions work best for her, at whatever time of day best fits her schedule, so long as she stays *within three grams* of each macro goal number each day.

It takes time and practice, but each day, she'll get better at "budgeting."

THE NERDY GAME OF TETRIS

As you just saw, macro tracking isn't some big, confusing dieting scheme. It's simply a matter of dividing your total goal calories into grams of carbs, fats, and protein, and aiming to hit those numbers each day.

Think of it this way: I give you one hundred dollars to spend on anything you want. The only rule is you must spend all one hundred dollars *today*. Tomorrow, you'll get a new one hundred dollars , but it doesn't roll over and you can't save it.

Without a budgeting plan, you might blow ninety-five dollars on breakfast and lunch. Now it's dinnertime and you're eyeing your five-dollar sandwich with disdain. The next day, the memory of that stale tuna on rye might lead you to overcompensate in the other direction. Now you hold onto every penny until 6:00 p.m., when you finally realize the day's more than half over, you haven't eaten or done anything all day, and you now have six hours to blow every cent. By the third day, you begin to understand how this works a bit better. You come up with a plan to spread your money out evenly throughout the day: ten dollars here, five dollars there, and so on. But then the fourth day hits. It's 10:00 a.m., and you find yourself standing in front of a life-size replica of Michelangelo from the Teenage Mutant Ninja Turtles. Clearly, you need this statue in your life. And, *oh happy day*, it's on sale! Fifty dollars for the embodiment of cool but rude?! That's a no-brainer.

But, wait.

That's half of your budget spent before noon! Making this investment means you'll need to be thrifty the rest of the day. Is it worth it? You decide it is, happily hand over your cash, strut down the street dragging your new favorite prized possession, and merrily budget the rest of your day, rejoicing in the decision to trade a bit of thriftiness for a treasured memento. You've learned how to budget for bigger purchases and still stay within your daily allotment.

This is exactly how macro tracking works.

We budget.

Instead of a one-hundred-dollar budget, we have a macro budget. Once we know our numbers, our daily allowance for each macro, we can eat the foods we love, so long as we stay within our budget. This ensures a balance of all macronutrients, *and*, this is a huge one for those of us sick of yo-yoing, it's not based on restriction. No foods are off-limits.

Because it's calculated mathematically, not guesswork, and because it allows for choice and isn't based on restriction, macro tracking is aligned with how we as human beings are designed, both physically and psychologically. We're not fighting against our human nature to avoid pain and seek pleasure; we're not forcing ourselves into a state of discomfort through restriction. We're actively giving ourselves choices and making decisions based on our individual goals and preferences.

I call macro tracking a Nerdy Game of Tetris because it's all about making things fit—in this case, the food we *choose* to eat. Just like our daily monetary budget, it takes time and practice to hit the numbers on the head. It takes tweaking and adjusting. With practice and consistency, it gets easier and easier, until it becomes a sustainable lifestyle.

Let's say Julianna's macro breakdown looked like this:

Total Calories: 1,552
Carbs: 189 grams
Fat: 44 grams
Protein: 100 grams

She would first enter these numbers into the "goal" portion of her app. From there, her job is to enter the food she eats each day, making adjustments to get closer and closer to hitting these numbers.

So, the first day, she tracks her breakfast:

2 whole eggs
1 slice whole wheat toast
2 tablespoons peanut butter

50 grams avocado

Her app shows her current macro totals from her meal as:

Total breakfast calories: 520

Carbs: 34 grams

Fat: 34 grams

Protein: 25 grams

Holy fat macros, Batman! Her fat macros are at 34 grams from breakfast alone, leaving her only 10 grams of fat for the rest of the day! This shows her that she might need to make some swaps. It *does not* mean peanut butter goes on the blacklist of restricted food. Rather, it means she may need to choose *between* the avocado or peanut butter tomorrow morning. Or maybe she decides to leave her breakfast as is and, just like your killer Ninja Turtle purchase, be stingy with eating fatty food for the rest of the day. The choice is hers. She has 44 grams of fat to "spend" each day, and how she spends them is up to her.

This is where the Nerdy Game of Tetris comes in. It's all about making things fit.

While the nutrition label on a food like olive oil will show one serving as:

Carbs: 0

Protein: 0

Fat: 14 grams

Most food will contain all three macros. Which means, just like adding a piece to the puzzle of Tetris, once you add the food, all three numbers adjust.

For example, an average serving of peanut butter contains:

Carbs: 8 grams

Protein: 7 grams

Fat: 16 grams

So, if you're looking to up your protein and you went to peanut butter because the jar claimed it was an "excellent source of protein," yes, you did get a few grams of protein, but you just added a whooole lotta fat to the mix as well.

It becomes a game of "fitting" your foods into your macros. I fully realize that "game" may seem like a stretch right now, but, I promise, it becomes fun, in the nerdiest way possible. As you see clearly what's in the food you're eating, you learn to make choices aligned with your goals to better fit your personal puzzle.

There are two beautiful things I love about this process:

1. **It's not based on restriction.** Love peanut butter? Eat peanut butter. Just make it fit your macros. Hate peanut butter? Don't eat it. Choose different fats for your macros. It's all about what *you* like to eat. Vegetarian, vegan, pescatarian, raw food, carnivore, whatever your preference, tracking macros works.
2. **You can plan ahead.** If I go out to eat, chances are I'm having pizza. On days where a big ol' slice of deliciousness is in my future, I'll plug it into my app first thing in the morning, before I've even brushed my teeth, let alone gone to the restaurant at dinnertime. That way, I can "budget" the rest of my day leading up to dinner, already having accounted for that meal.

Pizza no longer has to be a "cheat meal" or mean I've "ruined my diet." It means I made a choice to use a good amount of that day's macros on that one meal, and I'll make it fit by tweaking the rest of that day's meals.

Blammo! Nerdy Tetris.

Learning to "budget" for the foods you love means there are no longer "good" or "bad" foods. There are no longer "approved" foods and foods that "aren't" allowed. Giving yourself choice and flexibility, not living by restriction, is the key to making nutrition a sustainable lifestyle.

TRACKING AND PREPLANNING

It's 10:00 p.m. and Casey lays down in her bed for the night. She reaches for her phone to scroll through social media. In the middle of commenting on the third pit bulls cuddling video she's watched, she remembers that she hasn't tracked her macros from that day.

Going into her app, she racks her mind, desperately trying to remember everything she ate since breakfast. Considering she can barely remember if she locked the front door before getting into bed, thinking back to what she consumed at 6:00 a.m. when her brain was barely functioning is a bit of a challenge. Not completely sure that she's got everything, she plugs in what she can remember.

With a sinking feeling in her stomach, Casey sees that she's gone over her carbs by seventy-five grams. Turns out pancakes for breakfast, pasta for lunch, *and* pizza for dinner did not all fit into her macros. With a closer look, she realizes that, had she input her food as the day went on, she could have still had her pancakes and pasta but made a dinner choice with slightly fewer carbs and still been within her numbers.

Inputting your food as the day goes on allows you to adjust as needed. When you see a number creeping up, or one that's still low as it gets later in the day, you can adjust accordingly. When we wait to input at the end of the day like Casey, we not only run the risk of forgetting what we ate, but there's also no way to go back and undo what's already done.

You can also preplan the night before. This is especially useful if you meal prep, as you know exactly what you're bringing for meals the next day. It's also useful for going out to eat, as evidenced by my pizza example. The key with preplanning is to allow for flexibility. A day can be perfectly planned out in our app, with all our macros right in range. When the day starts, however, maybe we're not hungry for breakfast and don't want the full meal we planned out the night before. Maybe we're super hungry at lunch and want to eat more than we planned. Remember, we're playing the Nerdy Game of Tetris and it's all about making things fit. You can adjust for a smaller breakfast and eat more at lunch. You can eat more at lunch and snack less before dinner. Having a plan is a great way to set yourself up for success. Being flexible allows us to execute it realistically.

THE LEARNING PROCESS

If you've spent your entire life thus far buying lattes four out of seven days a week, hitting the "buy now" button without a second thought when shopping online, and putting bills on autopay so you can set it and forget it, expecting complete financial freedom in a matter of days, or even weeks, is setting yourself up for frustration.

It's the same with tracking macros.

If you've spent the majority of your life having no idea how many calories were coming in each day, let alone how many grams of carbs, fat, and protein, expecting yourself to nail your numbers right away is a recipe, pun intended, for frustration and giving up. Know that this takes time, practice, and tweaking. You'll get there. Using your mindset tools will help you through the learning curve until you get to a place where the new neural pathway is wired in, and macro tracking feels like second nature to you.

I say Nerdy Game of Tetris because that's what it is: *a game*. Make it fun. Enjoy the process. Best of all, winning at this game gets you more than a congratulatory message on a screen with a fun little jingle. It gets you control of your nutrition, and the way your body looks and feels, for the rest of your life.

That's a big freakin' deal.

Put in the Work

Today's a monumental day for you! Today we figure out *your* numbers, putting you on the path to making nutrition a sustainable lifestyle!

Let's go through the process together. Remember, if you start to feel overwhelmed, or if that caveman brain wants to talk you out of doing the work, use the mindset tools you've learned in this book. Recognize that it's Fear wanting to keep you in your comfort zone. Talk to yourself like a kindergartener. Put your trust in me. Use every tool you learned in this book and *keep going*. This *will* change your relationship with food for the rest of your life once you build the habit. You can do this.

Grab your journal and work through the sections below. Leave room, as you may want to come back to this process after a few weeks of consistently hitting your macros to see if any adjustments need to be made. Macros are never "one and done." As you give them time to work, you always want to be checking in with your energy level and your results and adjust as needed. You'll also want to adjust as your weight starts changing.

Use the formula from Chapter VIII to find your TDEE.

This is the only part of the process where I would suggest using an online calculator if you don't want to do the math. While you will find a plethora of macro calculators online, I don't recommend using them. A simple test of two of these calculators will show you why. They tend to spit out wildly different results resulting in, best case scenario, confusion, and, worst case scenario, the opposite result of what you're looking to accomplish. TDEE calculators tend to be more reliable, as the formula is more or less standard.

A free TDEE calculator is available to you on my website: www.MindStrongFitness.com/Becoming.

You can also use the formula below and do the work by hand:

For women:

655 + (4.35 × weight in pounds) + (4.7 × height in inches) − (4.7 × age in years) = Your BMR (Basal Metabolic Rate), the number of calories required to keep your body functioning *at rest*.

For men:

66 + (6.23 × weight in pounds) + (12.7 × height in inches) − (6.8 × age in years)

Then:

If you are sedentary and do not exercise, multiply your BMR by 1.2.

If you exercise lightly one to three times per week, multiply by 1.375.

Again, light exercise can mean lifting weights that don't cause you to make weird noises or going for jogs that get your heart going. It does not mean you powerwalk to Taco Bell one to three times a week.

If you exercise to the point of really breaking a sweat three to five days per week, multiply by 1.55.

For intense exercise six or seven days per week, multiply by 1.725.

Is your goal to maintain your current weight, gain, or lose?

If your goal is to maintain, you're done with this part! Your TDEE is the same as your total calories. Go on to the steps below.

If your goal is to gain, I suggest adding about 10–15 percent to your TDEE to start. You can continue to increase as needed, but start low, monitor how you feel, and adjust as needed.

If your goal is to lose, subtract 10–15 percent, being sure to not go below ten times your body weight. Remember, *sustainability is key*, so start where you're comfortable, knowing you can always adjust to be more aggressive down the road.

1. Write down your total calories based on your goal.
2. Protein: Take your body weight and multiply it by .8–1, depending on if you currently work out consistently and/or your average from the five days of tracking you've already done. If your goal is to build muscle from your work in the gym, lean toward the factor of 1. If you're not in the gym and/or your protein average is currently low, start at .8, knowing you can always come back and adjust. Write down your protein goal.
3. Fat: Take your body weight and multiply by .35–.45. If you prefer carbs over fat, stay toward .35. If your fat average was high in your five days of tracking, start at the .45 range, knowing you can always go back and adjust as your diet changes. Write down your fat goal.
4. Carbs: Now for some nerdy math. We need to figure out how many calories we have remaining. Write down your answers to these steps:
   a. Using your answer in #2 above, multiply your protein goal (in grams) by 4. This will give your calorie intake for protein, because 1 gram of protein equals 4 calories.
   b. Using your answer in #3 above, multiply your fat goal (in grams) by 9. This will give you your calorie intake for fat, because 1 gram of fat equals 9 calories.
   c. Now add together your totals from A and B.

d. Using your answer in #1 above, write down your total calories.

e. Take your answer from D and subtract your answer from C. This gives us your remaining calories.

f. Last step: Take your calories from E and divide by 4 (because 1 gram of carbs equals 4 calories). This number is your grams of carbs. If you get a decimal, round up or down according to the old middle school rule of .5 or above goes up, .4 or below goes down.

g. Write down your total grams of carbs.

Now, write down your personal starting macros:

- Total Calories:
- Protein:
- Fat:
- Carbs:

For example, Christine's TDEE is 1,864 calories. She wants to lose fat, so she subtracts 15 percent and comes up with a daily caloric intake of 1,584.

She currently works out and weighs 120 pounds, so she sets her protein at 120 grams (120 × 1).

She prefers carbs over fat, because she likes to fuel her workouts with the macronutrient her body goes to for energy first. So, she multiples her body weight, 120, by .35 and gets 42 grams of fat.

Now it's time for some nerdy math.

Since 1 gram of protein = 4 calories and Christine has 120 grams of protein, she has currently used 480 calories worth of protein (120 × 4).

Since 1 gram of fat = 9 calories and Christine has 42 grams of protein, she's used 378 calories on fat.

When we add up her protein calories plus her fat calories, we see that Christine has currently used 858 calories so far (480 protein + 378 fat).

Since her daily caloric intake is 1,584, she subtracts 1,584 − 858 (total used calories so far), and sees that she has 726 calories to be used in carbs.

One gram of carbs = 4 calories, so Christine divides 726/4, and gets 181.5, which she rounds up to 182 grams of carbs per day.

So, Christine's personal macros would look like this:

Total Calories Per Day: 1586
(I rounded up so our nerdy math is exact)

Protein: 120 grams

Fat: 42 grams

Carbs: 182 grams

We can check our numbers by ensuring our macros add up to our total calories:

---

120 (Protein)
+ 182 (Carbs)
= 302   **42** (Fat)
× 4*   **× 9****

| **1,208** | **+** | **378** | **=** | **1,586** Total Calories |

*because both protein and carbs are 4 calories per gram
**because one gram of fat is 9 calories

Go into your macro tracking app, find where you input "goals," and plug them in.

Note that some apps have a free version and a paid version. The free version on most will not allow you to type in exact numbers. They're limited to typing in your total calories and breaking down each macro by percentage. If you choose to use the free version, the tracking part works the same. You will just have to set your goals as close as possible and then refer back to your notes of your actual numbers until you have them memorized. If you want to avoid this, you can upgrade to the paid version of the app, which allows you to type in your exact numbers for each macro.

Remember to input your food as the day goes on. If you wait until the end of the day, it's already in your belly, and there's nothing we can do about it. Tracking as you go allows you to adjust your food choices as the day goes on, according to what you have left in your "budget."

Learning to track macros takes practice. We're building a new skill, and, as we learned from our work with habits and brain plasticity, that takes time, repetition, and consistency. You *can* do this. With practice, you *will* do this. Don't give up! Keep tracking, keep adjusting, and keep learning! Remember that embarking on any new journey opens the door for our caveman brain to run rampant and for Fear to sneak in. This process is the perfect opportunity for you to put your new tool bag of mindset techniques to use so you can master the Nerdy Game of Tetris!

CHAPTER XI

DAY ONE

"How to begin the journey? You need only to take the first step. When? There is always now."
—GEORGE LEONARD

I am so freakin' proud of you. We started this book with a few important steps to make a healthy lifestyle sustainable, and you've crushed each and every one:

1. **Start.** If you're here with me, you've not only started, but you're well on your way. That's massive. That shows you're ready for and dedicated to change.
2. **This isn't all in or all out.** Unless you found yourself *so* absorbed in this book that you read it cover to cover without getting up to pee, chances are life happened in-between chapters. And yet, here we are. You continued to come back. You did the exercises. *(If you didn't, go back and start now!)* You kept going. That's the key.
3. **Education.** You came here to learn how health and fitness work once and for all, to be empowered to do this for the rest of your life without the need for anyone else. Yes, you'll

continue to learn, grow, and up your game. Our goal was to acquire the tools needed to begin. And now you've got that.

You can do this. Change takes time and, most of all, conscious effort. But there is nothing in this life that you can't accomplish with education, time, and consistency.

You've now got the education.

Go put in the work.

Put in the Work

I don't know about you, but my bookshelf is filled with literally hundreds of books earmarked for exercises that I'll come back to "someday."

Most of those books have been sitting in the same condition for about five to fifteen years. In other words, someday never came. This explains why I have so many books on the same topic. If I had actually done the work suggested in the first book I bought, I wouldn't have needed to read, and subsequently ignore, the ten other books, all filled with similar information.

This stuff works when you put in the work. As the old saying goes, "Nothing changes if nothing changes."

So, let's make some changes.

This final Put in the Work takes into account every area of your life affected by the topics within this book. Remember, if our thoughts are affecting our feelings, which in turn affect our actions, which affect our results, which then lead us back to related thoughts, getting honest with ourselves about where we stand in each area shows us exactly where we need to put our focus and dig a little deeper.

If any of this brings up feelings of Fear, go back and read chapter VI on Fear. That chapter, and all chapters in this book, are intended to be a resource, yours to come back to for rereading as often as needed. As you make more and more progress in your new, empowered, healthy lifestyle, new fears will come up. That's when it's time to reread.

Mindset

Grab your journal. Close your eyes. Take a deep, calming breath. Picture yourself in the near future, living with abundant health, energy out the whazoo, and the body of your dreams. What thoughts just popped into your mind? How confident do you feel about achieving this?

Now, open your eyes and write down the most relevant answer from this list:

1. I won't do it. I never do. I'll probably just quit like I always do.
2. I want to do it, but it's tough to believe it's possible. I promised myself I will be all in from here on out, but I haven't done the work in the earlier chapters to understand how this works.
3. I feel hopeful but scared. I'm in, 100 percent, I've committed to a few first steps to get my momentum going, but I haven't put in all the work before, so I'm not quite sure what to do in some areas.
4. Hellllll yeah, that life is MINE FOR THE TAKING. I'm on my macro game, have a few first steps to get my momentum rolling, and am committed to never being "all in/all out" again!

Now, read your answer and write down your responses to these questions:

• How do you feel when you read this?
• What *actions* do you think these feelings will lead to?
• What will your results be?
• If you don't feel pumped up, ready to jump out of your seat and dive into your new, healthy, empowered lifestyle 100 percent, what action steps are you going to take to get your answer to "Hellllll yeah" above? Be specific.

All the tools you need are in this book. It may mean rereading a chapter for a mindset shift. It may mean pausing, breathing, and having a kindergarten convo with yourself. It may mean doing a Put in the Work that you earmarked earlier in this book. It may mean rereading some work you did over the course of this book. Write it all down. Set yourself up for success.

Thoughts-Feelings-Actions-Results

You now understand that your thoughts lead to the feelings you have, the actions those feelings lead you to take, and the results that come from those actions. Those actions, then, lead full circle back to the thoughts you think, and on and on the cycle goes. Taking an honest look at your life, which answer best describes your current Thoughts-Feelings-Actions-Results loop? Write it down.

- I don't know why my results in each area of life are what they are.
- I see how my actions get their results. I don't understand why my feelings and thoughts are affecting them.
- I've started to identify that my results in certain areas of my life are what they are, first and foremost, because of my thoughts. I'm paying attention whenever I feel something uncomfortable, tracing it back to my thoughts, and doing my best to reframe.
- I am 100 percent responsible for the results of my life. I know that a belief is a thought I've repeated over and over until I've accepted it as Truth, and I am responsible for my thoughts and beliefs about everything around me. By taking control of my thoughts, I can choose to feel feelings that serve me, take actions that serve me, get the results that serve me, and design the life that I dream of.

Read your answer and write down your responses to these questions:

- How do you feel when you read this?

- What *actions* do you think these feelings will lead to?
- What will your results be?
- Everything starts with your thoughts. How will you monitor where your thoughts are in a day and train your internal voice to be your best coach instead of your harshest critic?

This may mean rereading the Thoughts-Feelings-Actions-Results chapter, setting a reminder on your phone to check in with how you're feeling a few times a day, ensuring you're pausing to have kindergartener conversations anytime you catch that internal voice beating you up, or pausing, breathing, and checking in with your thoughts when you experience a feeling you don't like. Write it all down.

Daily Habits

Let's take a look at your current daily habits. Remember, the intention of this isn't to judge or be harsh on yourself. We want to clearly see *why* our life is the way it is and, most importantly, what we can do to improve the areas where we feel stuck. Don't filter. Don't overthink. What do your current daily habits look like? Write it down.

- My daily habits are based around everyone else. I don't have time to think about me.
- I want to change. I feel burned-out. I need some new habits.
- I've started implementing a few new habits to make sure I'm taking care of myself, but not as much as I'd like to be.
- I know that the way I can show up as my best self for those I love is by taking care of myself. My daily habits reflect the importance of making sure my health is a priority.

Read through your answer and then answer these questions:

- How do you feel when you read this?

- What *actions* do you think these feelings will lead to?
- What will your results be?
- What habits will you *consciously change* to ensure you love the life you're living? Remember, habits are rooted deep in our brain. They take conscious and consistent effort, so make sure the thoughts *and the feelings they bring* are strong enough to make them a priority.
- Write down every habit you're committed to changing and *how* you will ensure this conscious change remains a priority.

Fear

Fear is a huge topic. It's what can stop us from living the life of our dreams. As we read, it is only by redefining Fear that we can use it to our advantage rather than continuing on a path where it calls the shots and keeps us feeling stuck. How are you currently feeling about your relationship with Fear? Write it down.

- Fear runs my life.
- I don't always notice it, but I walk around with this feeling like I could be doing more. I'm pretty sure it's Fear holding me back.
- My Redefine Fear exercise helped me shine some serious light. I've released a lot of Fear and continue to identify it as it comes.
- Psssht, Fear?! He can kiss my squatting booty! Yeah, he creeps in, then I acknowledge him, thank him, and send him on his merry way! I've decided that *I'm* running the show now.

Read through your answer and then answer these questions:

- How do you feel when you read this?
- What *actions* do you think these feelings will lead to?
- What will your results be?
- Fear will always be there. It's biological. What's your action plan for dealing with it when it invariably arrives?

This could mean rereading chapter VI on Fear or doing the Redefine Fear exercise for various areas of life. I've done one for health and fitness, money, and relationships, all just as powerful each time. It could be a conversation you have, out loud or in your head, when you feel Fear, or a mantra you choose to repeat to remind yourself what fear is and what it is not. Write it all down.

Energy

Let's take a moment to get honest about your current state of energy. Remember, life is energy. We get back what we put forth. What are your feelings on your current energy level? As always, write it down.

- What's that? I constantly feel like I'm crashing.
- I make it through the day but dream of my couch the moment work ends and find it hard to get back up once I sit down.
- I'm noticing shifts in my energy. The positive results I'm seeing are giving me momentum to keep making changes.
- I am on FIIIIIRE! My energy is through the roof, and I'm reaping the benefits in my life.

Read your answer and write down your responses to these questions:

- How do you feel when you read this?
- What *actions* do you think these feelings will lead to?
- What will your results be?
- Because like attracts like, your current life is a direct reflection of the energy you put out into the world. What specific steps will you take to start raising your vibration?

This could include going back and rereading chapter VII, Life Is Energy, ensuring you're having kindergarten convos in your head each time that harsh voice creeps in, or journaling about your future self as if it's the current situation because we now know that your brain can't tell the difference. Write down the first steps you will take to start raising your vibration and living the life you dream of.

Eating for Your Goals

Calories are energy. What we put in is what fuels our body. How are you feeling about your relationship with food right now? What thoughts come to mind when you think about eating for your goals? Write it down in your journal.

- It's too hard. I've tried and failed too many times.
- I would like to, but when I get hungry, I grab whatever's around me. I don't have the self-control for this.
- It sounds challenging, but if I plan ahead and ensure I always have food with me so I can stay on track the majority of the time, I'll be successful.
- Piece of cake, pun intended. I know how great I'll feel when I do it, so momentum will keep me going.

Now, read your answer and write down your responses to these questions:

- How do you feel when you read this?
- What *actions* do you think these feelings will lead to?
- What will your results be?
- What can you think or do to reframe your thoughts and, by extension, your actions about eating for your goals? Again, be specific. It could be anything from an internal convo, to creating food shopping lists, to meal planning. Write it all down.

Macros

Tracking macros is how we redefine our relationship with food. We learn to eat for our goals in a way that's aligned with both science and psychology. How are you currently feeling about your journey into the world of macros? Write down your answer in your journal.

- I don't understand what a macro is or why tracking macros can help.
- I get it, but it seems like a lot of work.
- I've started but haven't fully committed. Something's holding me back.
- I'm in! I've figured out my numbers, been tracking, and am committed to the process, knowing it's sustainable because it's not based on restriction. I feel free!

Read your answer and respond to the questions below:

- How do you feel when you read this?
- What *actions* do you think these feelings will lead to?
- What will your results be?
- What can you think or do to reframe your thoughts and, by extension, your actions about tracking macros? It could be anything from an internal convo, to rereading the macro chapters, to Putting in the Work on those chapters. Be specific and *go do it!*

At the start of this book, you wrote down a declaration, agreeing to never again be all in or all out. You committed to being in.

You'll have days where you crush it. You'll have days where you kinda suck at this. You'll have days you hit personal records in the gym, and days where tying your shoes feels like a lot of work. Some days you'll hit your macros spot-on, some days you'll wonder if the Krispy Kreme fairy shoved four donuts in your mouth while you were sleeping because there's no way in hell you actually ate that much for breakfast without realizing it.

It doesn't matter.

You're in.

You get back on.

You keep going.

You've now got the education.

All that's left are time and consistency.

You can do that.

ADDITIONAL RESOURCES

My work in this world is to help you unleash your most empowered life, not by the fleeting motivation of passively reading a book but by *taking the actionable steps* outlined here, as well as supporting you as you continue to grow and evolve on your health and fitness journey.

To further support you, you'll find all the resources mentioned throughout the book on my website, www.MindStrongFitness. com/Becoming, including:

- TDEE calculator
- Simple versus complex carb cheat sheet
- Suggested fat sources
- Suggested protein sources
- Suggested apps for macro tracking
- Supplement guide
- Where to start in the gym
- And much more!

As with everything in life, the more you develop and level up, the more questions you will have. For this reason, you will also find a

FAQ section on my website addressing common questions that often arise on this journey.

As you know by now, I am a huge fan of momentum. Your journey starts here, with the work you did in this book. As that momentum grows, you may hit a point where you're ready to take your health and fitness to the next level. Information on my online coaching programs can also be found on my website, www. MindStrongFitness.com/Becoming.

ACKNOWLEDGMENTS

I used to joke that if I ever wrote a book, it would be called *Everything I Need to Know About Life, I Learned from Weight Training*. I now realize that another book would be appropriate: *Everything I Need to Know About Life, I Learned from Writing a Book*. At the top of that list would be the value of having loving, supportive people around you.

I can't imagine, nor would I want to experience, the writing process without the guidance, support, and love from everyone around me, especially the following people:

My parents, for supporting me from my Scotty days to present day.

Jason, for understanding what the Freiman mindset means.

My MindStrong Fam. You are my inspiration.

Kathy, Janin, Liz, Susan, and Emi for your time, energy, and insight.

Meredith, my sounding board in both business and life.

Victor, my Gladiator brother.

Marie, for your expertise, support, and no-BS approach to book coaching.

Tracy, for your unyielding guidance and love, and for teaching me what it means to redefine fear.

Amanda, thank you for your support, always.

Charlie, for loaning your momma to the world while she wrote and for providing much-needed end-of-the-night cuddles.

ABOUT THE AUTHOR

Originally from NYC, Rachel Freiman's path to fitness was an odd one.

After attending the Interlochen Arts Academy and various music colleges, Rachel earned her bachelor's degree in music education and her master's degree in jazz performance. She went on to be a freelance jazz musician in NYC for over ten years, before moving to Florida for a calmer life of teaching middle school music. This is where Rachel discovered both her passion for teaching and the need to lift heavy shit at the end of a long school day.

The more she went to the gym, the more people started coming with her, looking for friendly guidance on how to feel their best. It soon became clear that Rachel's true zone of genius wasn't in teaching a single subject matter but in teaching people how to ignite their inner spark and live their healthiest, most fulfilled life.

This passion for helping people unleash their badassiest self led to the birth of MindStrong Fitness.

Rachel now lives in Arizona with her puppy, Charlie. When she's not in the gym, Rachel enjoys exploring the world, snuggling with Charlie, eating, and thinking about the next time she'll be eating.

REFERENCES

1   Christina Steindl et al., "Understanding Psychological Reactance: New Developments and Findings," *Zeitschrift für Psychologie* 223, no. 4 (2015): 205-214, https://doi.org/10.1027/2151-2604/a000222.

2   Roy F. Baumeister et al., "Ego Depletion: Is the Active Self a Limited Resource?" *Journal of Personality and Social Psychology* 74, no. 5 (1998): 1252-1265.

3   Marianne Szegedy-Maszak, "Mysteries of the Mind," *U.S. News & World Report*, February 28, 2005, 52-4, 57-8, 60-1, PubMed PMID: 15765847.

4   Scott Bea, "How to Turn Your Negative Thinking Around," October 3, 2019, https://health.clevelandclinic.org/turn-around-negative-thinking/.

5   Nicolò F. Bernardi et al., "Mental Practice Promotes Motor Anticipation: Evidence from Skilled Music Performance," *Frontiers in Human Neuroscience* 7 (2013): 451, https://doi.org/10.3389/fnhum.2013.00451.

6   Tom Hughes, "The Power of Thoughts," *Brian Mackenzie's Successful Coaching*, 2006, 8-9.

7   Donald O. Hebb, *The Organization of Behavior* (New York: Wiley & Sons, 1949).

8   Roy F. Baumeister et al., "Bad Is Stronger Than Good," *Review of General Psychology* 5 (2001): 323-370, https://doi.org/10.1037//1089-2680.5.4.323.

9   Much of the Fear work in this book comes from my personal privilege of working with mindset coach Tracy Litt, author of *Worthy Human*, Lioncrest Publishing, 2019.

10 "OpenStax, Atoms, Isotopes, Ions, and Molecules: The Building Blocks," OpenStax CNX, Feb 3, 2015, http://cnx.org/contents/be8818d0-2dba-4bf3-859a-737c25fb2c99@@12.

11 The *only* exception to this is when you are brand new to lifting weights *and* extremely overweight. Studies have shown that people who are obese and start a regular weightlifting routine will experience a *brief* period of time where their body can access energy stores and convert it to muscle. This doesn't mean casually walking three blocks to Mickey D's while holding two-pound dumbbells. It means you're pushing your muscles to lift heavier weights than they can consistently do, four to five days a week, while in a caloric deficit. Even so, *brief* is the key word here. In time, even the population who fit in this category will be back to the hard and fast rule of muscle growth.

12 Kristin Fischer, "Here Are the Worst Side Effects of the Keto Diet," updated July 24, 2018, Healthline, https://www.healthline.com/health-news/worst-side-effects-of-the-keto-diet.

13 Julia Ries, "Yes, Keto Diarrhea Is a Thing: How the Popular Diet Can Disrupt Digestion," September 20, 2018, Healthline, https://www.healthline.com/health-news/how-the-keto-diet-can-wreak-havoc-on-your-gi-system.

14 Maciej Banach, "Caution against Cutting Down on Carbohydrates," ESC Congress News 2018—Munich, Germany, European Society of Cardiology, August 28, 2018, https://www.escardio.org/Congresses-&-Events/ESC-Congress/Congress-resources/Congress-news/caution-against-cutting-down-on-carbohydrates.

15 Chia-Yu Chang, Der-Shin Ke, and Jen-Yin Chen, "Essential Fatty Acids and Human Brain," *Acta Neurol Taiwan* 18, no. 4 (2009): 231–41, PubMed PMID: 20329590.

16 Chang, Ke, and Chen, "Essential Fatty Acids and Human Brain," 231–41.

17 Heysook Yoon et al., "Interplay between Exercise and Dietary Fat Modulates Myelinogenesis in the Central Nervous System," *Biochimica et Biophysica Acta (BBA)—Molecular Basis of Disease* 1862, no. 4 (2016): 545–555, https://doi.org/10.1016/j.bbadis.2016.01.019.